MRI in Practice

Second edition

CATHERINE WESTBROOK MSc, DCR, CTC
Education and Research Co-ordinator in MRI
University of Oxford

AND

CAROLYN KAUT RT,(R),(MR)
Director, Technologist Continuing Education Programme
Hospital University of Pennsylvania

Mic info.com

Blackwell
Science

© 1993, 1998 by Blackwell Science Ltd,
a Blackwell Publishing Company

Editorial Offices:
Blackwell Science Ltd, 9600 Garsington Road, Oxford OX4 2DQ, UK
   Tel: +44 (0)1865 776868
Blackwell Publishing Inc., 350 Main Street, Malden, MA 02148-5020, USA
   Tel: +1 781 388 8250
Blackwell Science Asia Pty, 550 Swanston Street, Carlton, Victoria 3053, Australia
   Tel: +61 (0)3 8359 1011

First published 1993
Reprinted 1994 (four times), 1995
Second edition published 1998
Reprinted 1999 (twice), 2000, 2001, 2002, 2003 (twice)

Library of Congress Cataloging-in-Publication Data
Westbrook, Catherine.
    MRI in practice/Catherine Westbrook
and Carolyn Kaut.—2nd ed.
       p.   cm.
    Includes bibliographical references and
index.
    ISBN 0-632-04205-2 (pbk.)
    1. Magnetic resonance imaging.
I. Kaut, Carolyn.   II. Title.
    [DNLM: 1. Magnetic Resonance
Imaging—methods.   2. Magnetic
Resonance Imaging—instrumentation.
WN 185 W523m   1998]
RC78.7.N83W48   1998
616.07′548—dc21
DNLM/DLC
for Library of Congress   97-45782
                                                                              CIP

ISBN 0–632–04205–2

A catalogue record for this title is available from the British Library

Set in 10/12pt Souvenir
by DP Photosetting, Aylesbury, Bucks
Printed and bound in Great Britain using acid-free
paper by MPG Books Ltd, Bodmin, Cornwall

For further information on Blackwell Publishing,
visit our website:
www.blackwellpublishing.com

Contents

Foreword

Dr Stephen Golding, Lecturer in Radiology, University of Oxford

The progress of magnetic resonance imaging (MRI) as a clinical tool has been extraordinary, out-stripping the rate of development of any other imaging technique. This speed of growth is a testimony to its clinical significance. Medical imaging specialists and their clinical colleagues have not been slow to grasp the advantages of an investigation which produces clear anatomical display in any plane, with no radiation risk to the patient, and with a tissue discrimination unrivalled by any other imaging technique. This process has accelerated rather than achieving a plateau and new clinical applications are constantly being defined.

Any new imaging technique brings with it an educational need, which in the case of MRI, is intense. The underlying technology is particularly complex and a working knowledge of it is essential to good practice. A case in point is fast imaging, which promises to change radically many of our diagnostic approaches. The radiologist, therefore, needs the support of technologists who are not only capable but also well informed to a degree not required in other radiological work; MRI is without doubt the modality where the changing dynamics of the technology and applications create our greatest challenges for continuing education.

The success of the first edition of this book is not surprising, considering the need and the fact that it was written not by scientists or radiologists for technologists, but by two technologists both actively involved in MRI, not only in clinical imaging but also in teaching their art to others. It is no surprise that a second edition has proved necessary so soon after the first and I welcome the new edition in the confidence that it will prove as valuable to readers as did its predecessor.

Preface

Since the first edition of *MRI in Practice* was published in 1993, its popularity has far outweighed even our most optimistic expectations. It is now considered an essential text for many MRI courses including the registry exam in the US and for post-graduate MRI programmes in the UK. A unique aspect of *MRI in Practice* is that it has crossed many boundaries that are not often traversed by other publications. Firstly, it is read on both sides of the Atlantic which is due, in part, to the dual nationality of the authors and secondly, it is not only popular with technologists and radiographers, but with many other professionals as well, including radiologists and medical students.

The success of *MRI in Practice* mainly lies in its clarity and logicality. It may not be physics in its purest form, but it clearly provides clinical MR practitioners relevant information at the right level. Developments in MRI happen at an astonishing rate and it is virtually impossible for a book to keep pace. In some respects physics is timeless, but new pulse sequences and hardware developments have increased the applications of MR substantially and it is therefore essential that a text such as this is constantly reviewed. In some respects updating a book such as *MRI in Practice* is a bit like painting the Golden Gate Bridge – no sooner have you finished one edition, a newer version is required!

In this, the second edition, you will find a new chapter on advanced techniques which discusses hardware and software developments and how they have opened up new applications. These include new abdominal applications, functional imaging and perfusion and diffusion studies. We have also expanded the sections on K space and pulse sequences to enable the reader to understand the concepts that underpin the new developments. Although expanded, we have tried to keep the explanations clear and simple. This edition isn't just about new applications however, we have also gone back to basics and overhauled the first chapter on basic principles. This now includes some quantum concepts which, we hope, has improved the clarity of this section.

There is no doubt that clinical MR practitioners require a book like *MRI in Practice* to help them understand why we do what we do. We hope that it will continue to serve this purpose and that it remains as popular as ever.

Catherine Westbrook
Carolyn Kaut

Acknowledgements

We continue to be extremely grateful to all those colleagues and family members who have supported us both professionally and personally and who continue to encourage us. Thank you. Without you, all this would never have been possible.

In addition to those mentioned in the first edition, I would like to especially thank several people; my husband Jon for sticking with it when I didn't deserve it; to Stephen Golding, Chris Kendell, Peter Sharpe and Liz Warren who I sincerely call my friends and to the world's most perfect children to which there has been another addition since last time. Madeleine, you are the light of my life.

CW

First, always I need to thank God for allowing the opportunity to begin such a project and providing the insight to complete it. Secondly, I need to thank my husband whose support and patience seem to go unnoticed . . . Scott, I do notice! Furthermore, I could not have got anywhere in MR without the help of my outsource partner and bestest buddy, Bill Faulkner. Finally, I could not even think of completing any MR publications without the full support of all the MR Technologists, Fellows, Staff and even the Tech interns at the University of Pennsylvania. Most of those were guys mentioned in the first edition and this time I need to add Suzie Brown, Glenn Ferrick and Dave Flint who are always there when I need them. Many thanks and love to all!

CK

Chapter 1   Basic Principles

Introduction

The basic principles of magnetic resonance imaging (MRI) form the foundation for further understanding of this complex subject. It is therefore, important that these ideas are fully grasped before continuing on to more complicated areas. There are essentially two ways of explaining the fundamentals of MRI; classically and via quantum physics. Any discussion requires both and so we have attempted to integrate the two versions. Within this chapter the properties of atoms and their interactions with magnetic fields, excitation and relaxation are discussed.

Atomic structure

The atom consists of a central nucleus and orbiting electrons (Fig. 1.1). The nucleus contains nucleons which are subdivided into protons and neutrons; protons are positively charged, neutrons have no net charge, and electrons are negatively charged. The *atomic number* is the sum of the protons in the nucleus, and the *mass number* is the sum of the protons and neutrons in the nucleus.

The atom is electrically stable if the number of negatively charged electrons orbiting the nucleus equals the number of positively charged protons in the nucleus. Atoms that are electrically unstable due to a deficit, or an excess number of electrons, are called *ions*.

Motion within the atom

Three types of motion are present within the atom (Fig. 1.2). These are:

(1) electrons spinning on their own axis,
(2) electrons orbiting the nucleus,
(3) the nucleus itself spinning about its own axis.

1

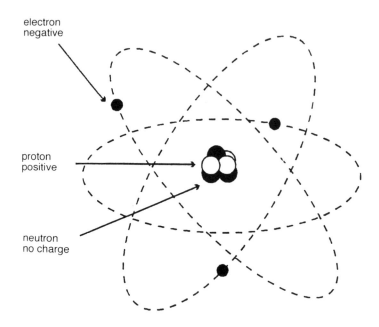

electron
negative

proton
positive

neutron
no charge

Fig. 1.1 The atom.

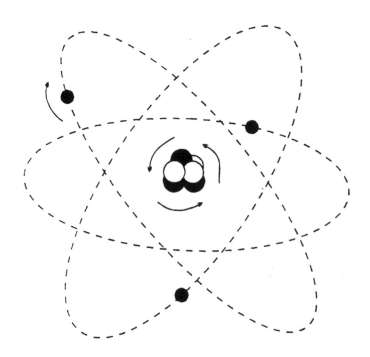

Fig. 1.2 Motion of particles in
the atom.

The principles of MRI rely on the spinning motion of specific nuclei present in biological tissues. These are known as *MR active* nuclei.

MR active nuclei

MR active nuclei are characterised by their tendency to align their axis of rotation to an applied magnetic field. Due to the laws of electromagnetic induction, nuclei that have a net charge and are spinning acquire a magnetic moment and are able to align with an external magnetic field. This occurs if the mass number is odd, i.e. there is either an even number of neutrons and an odd number of protons or vice versa. The process of this interaction is *angular momentum* or *spin*.

Important examples of MR active nuclei, together with their mass numbers are listed below:

hydrogen   1
carbon   13
nitrogen   15
oxygen   17
fluorine   19
sodium   23
phosphorus 31

Although neutrons have no net charge, their subatomic particles are not evenly arranged over the surface of the neutron and this imbalance enables the nucleus in which the neutron is situated to be MR active as long as the mass number is odd. Alignment can be measured as the total of the nuclear magnetic moments and is expressed as a vector sum. The strength of the total magnetic moment is specific to every nucleus and determines the sensitivity to magnetic resonance.

The hydrogen nucleus

The hydrogen nucleus is the MR active nucleus used in clinical MRI. The hydrogen nucleus contains a single proton (atomic and mass number 1). It is used because it is very abundant in the human body, and because its solitary proton gives it a relatively large magnetic moment.

The hydrogen nucleus as a magnet

The laws of electromagnetism state that a magnetic field is created when a charged particle moves. The hydrogen nucleus contains one positively charged proton that spins, i.e. it moves. Therefore the hydrogen nucleus has a magnetic field induced around it, and acts as a small magnet.

The magnet of each hydrogen nucleus has in effect a north and a south

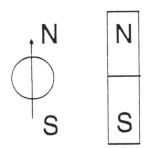

Fig. 1.3 The magnetic moment of the hydrogen nucleus.

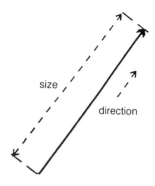

Fig. 1.4 The magnetic vector.

pole of equal strength. The north/south axis of each nucleus is represented by a *magnetic moment* (Fig. 1.3). The magnetic moment of each nucleus has vector properties, i.e. it has size and direction and is denoted by an arrow. The direction of the vector designates the direction of the magnetic moment, and the length of the vector designates the size of the magnetic moment as in Fig. 1.4.

Alignment

In the absence of an applied magnetic field the magnetic moments of the hydrogen nuclei are randomly orientated. When placed in a strong static external magnetic field however, the magnetic moments of the hydrogen nuclei align with this magnetic field (Fig. 1.5). Some of the hydrogen nuclei align parallel with the magnetic field (in the same direction), whereas a smaller number of the nuclei align anti-parallel to the magnetic field (in the opposite direction) as in Fig. 1.7.

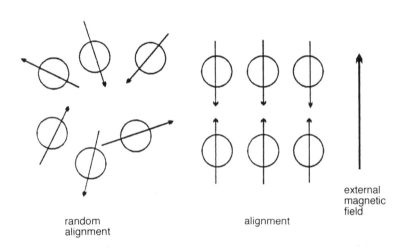

random
alignment

alignment

external
magnetic
field

Fig. 1.5 Alignment to the external field.

no external
field

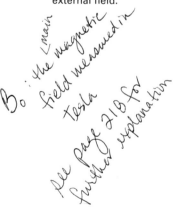

B_0 : the main magnetic field measured in Tesla. See page 21B for further explanation

Quantum physics describes the properties of electromagnetic radiation in terms of discrete quantities of energy rather than as waves (classical theory). Applying quantum physics to MRI, hydrogen nuclei only possess two energy states or populations – low and high (Fig. 1.6). Low energy nuclei align their magnetic moments parallel to the external field and are termed *spin up* nuclei. High energy nuclei align their magnetic moments in the anti-parallel direction and are termed *spin down* nuclei. Note that it is the *magnetic moments* of the hydrogen nuclei that align with B_0 and that they are only capable of aligning in one of two directions – parallel or anti-parallel to B_0.

The factors affecting which hydrogen nuclei align parallel and which align anti-parallel are determined by the strength of the external magnetic

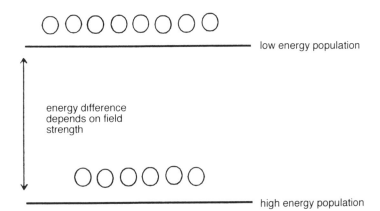

low energy population

energy difference
depends on field
strength

high energy population

Fig. 1.6 The two energy populations of hydrogen.

field and the thermal energy level of the nuclei. Low thermal energy nuclei do not possess enough energy to oppose the magnetic field in the anti-parallel direction. High thermal energy nuclei however, do possess enough energy to oppose this field, and as the strength of the magnetic field increases, fewer nuclei have enough energy to do so. The thermal energy of a nucleus is determined by the temperature of the patient. In clinical applications this cannot be significantly altered and so the emphasis is towards stronger magnetic fields.

In thermal equilibrium there are always fewer high energy nuclei than low energy nuclei therefore the magnetic moments of the nuclei aligned parallel to the magnetic field cancel out the smaller number of magnetic moments aligned anti-parallel. As there is a larger number aligned parallel, there is always a small excess in this direction that produces a net magnetic moment (Fig. 1.7). Other MR active nuclei also align to the magnetic field and produce their own small net magnetic moments. These magnetic moments are not used in clinical MRI because they do not exist in enough abundance in the body to be imaged adequately as their net magnetic moments are very small. However, with RF (radio frequency) coils tuned to the appropriate frequency and with adequate B_0 homogeneity it is possible to image other MR active nuclei. The net magnetic moment of hydrogen however, produces a significant magnetic vector that is used in clinical MRI.

- The magnetic moment of hydrogen is called the *net magnetisation vector (NMV)*.
- The static external magnetic field is called B_0.
- The interaction of the NMV with B_0 is the basis of MRI.
- The unit of B_0 is tesla or gauss. 1 tesla (T) is the equivalent of 10 000 gauss (G).

When a patient is placed in the bore of the magnet, the hydrogen nuclei within the patient align parallel and anti-parallel to B_0. A small excess of hydrogen nuclei line up parallel to B_0 and constitute the NMV of the patient (Fig. 1.7). The energy difference between the two populations

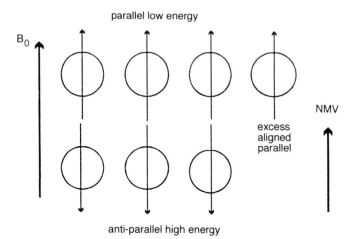

Fig. 1.7 The Net Magnetisation Vector (NMV).

increases as B_0 increases. Therefore at high field strengths fewer nuclei have enough energy to join the high energy population. This means that the magnitude of the NMV is larger at high field strengths than low field strengths, resulting in improved signal.

Precession

Each hydrogen nucleus that makes up the NMV is spinning on its axis as in Fig. 1.8. The influence of B_0 produces an additional spin, or wobble of the NMV around B_0. This secondary spin is called *precession* and causes the magnetic moments to follow a circular path around B_0. This path is called the *precessional path* and the speed at which the NMV wobbles around B_0 is called the *precessional frequency*. The unit of precessional frequency is megahertz (MHz) whereby 1 Hz is 1 cycle per second and 1 MHz is 1 million cycles per second.

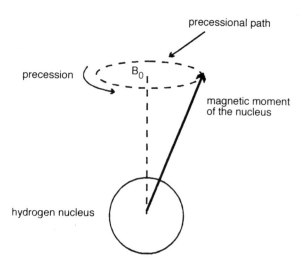

Fig. 1.8 Precession.

Combining Fig. 1.8 with what we now know about quantum physics, it is possible to appreciate that there are two populations of hydrogen nuclei – some high energy, spin down nuclei and a greater number of low energy, spin up hydrogen nuclei. The magnetic moments of all these nuclei precess around B_0 on a circular precessional path (Fig. 1.9).

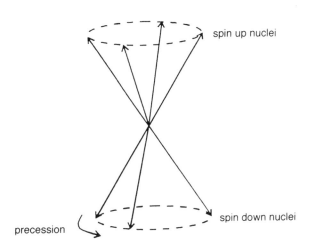

Fig. 1.9 Precession of the spin up and spin down populations.

The Larmor equation

The value of the precessional frequency is governed by the Larmor equation. The Larmor equation states that:

the precessional frequency $(\omega_0) = B_0 \times \gamma$

where B_0 is the magnetic field strength of the magnet, and
   γ is the gyro-magnetic ratio. The gyro-magnetic ratio expresses the relationship between the angular momentum and the magnetic moment of each MR active nucleus. It is constant and is expressed as the precessional frequency of a specific MR active nucleus at 1.0 T. The unit of the gyro-magnetic ratio is therefore MHz/T.

The gyro-magnetic ratio of hydrogen is 42.57 MHz/T. Other MR active nuclei have different gyro-magnetic ratios, and therefore have different precessional frequencies at the same field strength. In addition, hydrogen has a different precessional frequency at different field strengths. For example:

at 1.5 T the precessional frequency of hydrogen is 63.86 MHz
   (42.57 MHz × 1.5 T),
at 1.0 T the precessional frequency of hydrogen is 42.57 MHz
   (42.57 MHz × 1.0 T),
at 0.5 T the precessional frequency of hydrogen is 21.28 MHz
   (42.57 MHz × 0.5 T).

The precessional frequency is often called the *Larmor frequency*, because it is determined by the Larmor equation. As the gyro-magnetic ratio is a constant of proportionality, B_0 is proportional to the Larmor frequency. Therefore if B_0 increases, the Larmor frequency increases and vice versa.

Resonance

Resonance is a phenomenon that occurs when an object is exposed to an oscillating perturbation that has a frequency close to its own natural frequency of oscillation. When a nucleus is exposed to an external perturbation that has an oscillation similar to its own natural frequency, the nucleus gains energy from the external force. The nucleus gains energy and resonates if the energy is delivered at exactly its precessional frequency. If energy is delivered at a different frequency to that of the Larmor frequency of the nucleus, resonance does not occur.

Energy at the precessional frequency of hydrogen at all field strengths in clinical MRI corresponds to the radio frequency (RF) band of the electromagnetic spectrum (Fig. 1.10). For resonance of hydrogen to occur, an RF pulse of energy at exactly the Larmor frequency of the hydrogen NMV, must be applied. Other MR active nuclei that have aligned with B_0 do not resonate, because their precessional frequencies are different to that of hydrogen. The application of an RF pulse that causes resonance to occur is termed *excitation*. This absorption of energy causes an increase in the number of spin down hydrogen nuclei populations as some of the

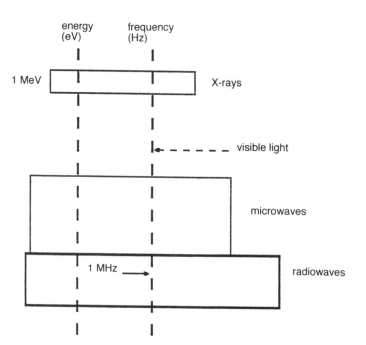

Fig. 1.10 The electromagnetic spectrum.

spin up nuclei gain energy via resonance and become high energy nuclei (Fig. 1.11). The energy difference between the two populations corresponds to the energy required to produce resonance via excitation. As the field strength increases, the energy difference between the two populations also increases so that more energy (higher frequencies) are required to produce resonance.

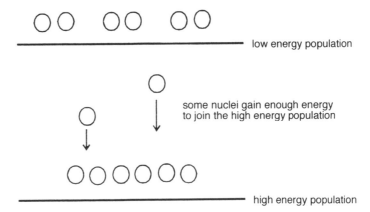

low energy population

some nuclei gain enough energy to join the high energy population

high energy population

Fig. 1.11 Energy transfer during excitation.

The results of resonance

The first result of resonance is that the NMV moves out of alignment away from B_0. The angle to which the NMV moves out of alignment is called the *flip angle* (Fig. 1.12). The magnitude of the flip angle depends upon the amplitude and duration of the RF pulse. Usually the flip angle is 90°, i.e. the NMV is given enough energy by the RF pulse to move through 90° relative to B_0.

- B_0 is now termed the *longitudinal axis/plane*.
- The plane at 90° to B_0 is termed the *transverse plane*.

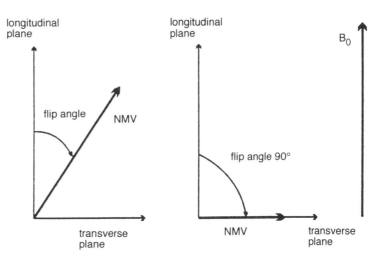

longitudinal plane

flip angle NMV

transverse plane

longitudinal plane

B_0

flip angle 90°

NMV transverse plane

Fig. 1.12 The flip angle. What flip angle will give the maximum transverse magnetisation?

With a flip angle of 90° the nuclei are given sufficient energy so that the longitudinal NMV is completely transferred into a transverse NMV. This transverse NMV rotates in the transverse plane at the Larmor frequency.

The second result of resonance is that the magnetic moments of the hydrogen nuclei within the transverse NMV move into phase with each other. *Phase* is the position of each magnetic moment on the precessional path around B_0. Magnetic moments that are *in phase*, are in the same place on the precessional path around B_0 at any given time, whereas magnetic moments that are *out of phase*, are not in the same place on the precessional path. When resonance occurs, all the magnetic moments move to the same position on the precessional path and are then in phase (Fig. 1.13).

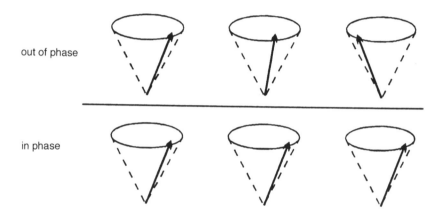

out of phase

in phase

Fig. 1.13 Phase of magnetic moments around their precessional path.

- For resonance of hydrogen to occur, RF at exactly the Larmor frequency of hydrogen must be applied.
- The result of resonance is an NMV in the transverse plane that is in phase.
- This NMV precesses in the transverse plane at the Larmor frequency.

The MR signal

As a result of resonance, the NMV is precessing in phase in the transverse plane. Faraday's laws of induction state that if a receiver coil or any conductive loop is placed in the area of a moving magnetic field, i.e. the NMV precessing in the transverse plane, a voltage is induced in this receiver coil. Signal is produced when coherent (in phase) magnetisation cuts across the coil. Therefore the moving NMV produces magnetic field fluctuations inside the coil. As the NMV precesses at the Larmor frequency in the transverse plane, a voltage is induced in the coil. This voltage constitutes the *MR signal*. The frequency of the signal is the same as the Larmor frequency – the magnitude of the signal depends on the amount of magnetisation present in the transverse plane. Why would you expect the MR signal in Fig. 1.14 to be alternating?

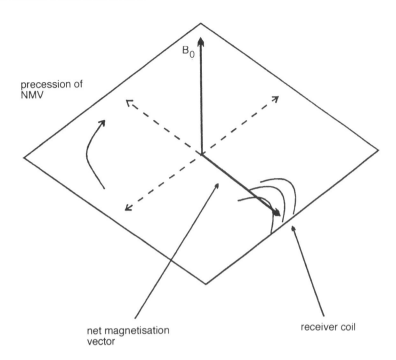

B_0

precession of
NMV

Fig. 1.14 Why would you
expect the MR signal to be
alternating?

net magnetisation
vector

receiver coil

The free induction decay signal (FID)

When the RF pulse is switched off, the NMV is again influenced by B_0 and
it tries to realign with it. In order to do so, the NMV must lose the energy
given to it by the RF pulse. The process by which the NMV loses this
energy is called *relaxation*. As relaxation occurs, the NMV returns to
realign with B_0.

- The amount of magnetisation in the longitudinal plane gradually
  increases – this is called *recovery*.

and at the same time but independently

- The amount of magnetisation in the transverse plane gradually
  decreases – this is called *decay*.

As the magnitude of transverse magnetisation decreases, so does the
magnitude of the voltage induced in the receiver coil. The induction in
reduced signal is called the *free induction decay (FID)* signal.

Relaxation

During relaxation the NMV gives up absorped RF energy and returns to
B_0. At the same time but independently the magnetic moments of the

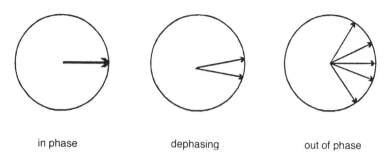

Fig. 1.15 Looking down on to the transverse plane ... dephasing.

in phase   dephasing   out of phase

NMV lose transverse magnetisation due to dephasing (Fig. 1.15). Relaxation results in recovery of magnetisation in the longitudinal plane and decay of magnetisation in the transverse plane.

- The recovery of longitudinal magnetisation is caused by a process termed *T1 recovery*.
- The decay of transverse magnetisation is caused by a process termed *T2 decay*.

T1 recovery

T1 recovery is caused by the nuclei giving up their energy to the surrounding environment or lattice, and it is often termed *spin lattice relaxation*. Energy released to the surrounding lattice causes nuclei to recover their longitudinal magnetisation (magnetisation in the longitudinal plane). The rate of recovery is an exponential process, with a recovery time constant called T1. This is the time it takes 63% of the longitudinal magnetisation to recover in the tissue (Fig. 1.16).

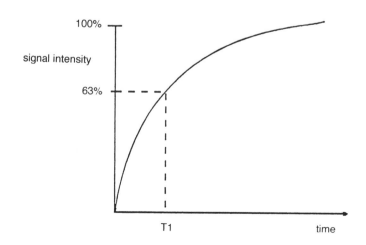

Fig. 1.16 The T1 recovery curve.

T2 decay

T2 decay is caused by nuclei exchanging energy with neighbouring nuclei. The energy exchange is caused by the magnetic fields of each nucleus interacting with its neighbour. It is often termed *spin spin relaxation* and results in a decay or loss of transverse magnetisation, (magnetisation in the transverse plane). The rate of decay is also an exponential process, so that the T2 relaxation time of a tissue is its time constant of decay. It is the time it takes 63% of the transverse magnetisation to be lost (Fig. 1.17).

- T1 relaxation results in the recovery of longitudinal magnetisation due to energy dissipation to the surrounding lattice.
- T2 relaxation results in the loss of transverse magnetisation due to interactions between the magnetic fields of adjacent nuclei.
- A signal or voltage is only induced in the receiver coil if there is magnetisation in the transverse plane, that is in phase (Fig. 1.18).

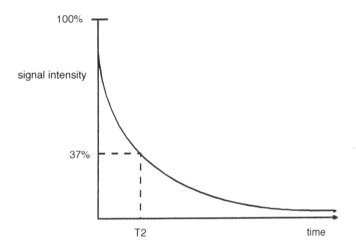

Fig. 1.17 The T2 decay curve.

LEARNING POINT

The NMV is a vector quantity. It is created by two components at 90° to each other. These two components are magnetisation in the longitudinal plane and magnetisation in the transverse plane (Fig. 1.19). Before resonance, there is full longitudinal magnetisation parallel to B_0. After the application of the RF pulse, the NMV is flipped fully into the transverse plane (assuming sufficient energy is applied). There is now full transverse magnetisation and zero longitudinal magnetisation.

Once the RF pulse is removed, the NMV recovers. As this occurs, the longitudinal component of magnetisation grows again, while the transverse component decreases. As the received signal amplitude is related to the magnitude of the transverse component, the signal in the coil decays as relaxation takes place.

The magnitude and timing of the RF pulses form the basis of MRI and are now discussed in more detail.

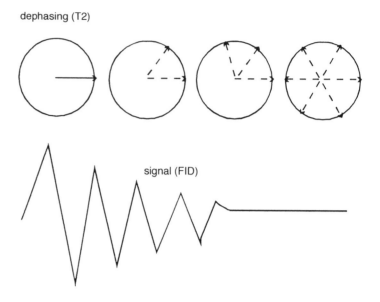

dephasing (T2)

signal (FID)

Fig. 1.18 Dephasing of the FID.

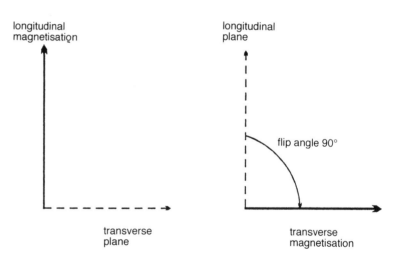

longitudinal magnetisation

transverse plane

longitudinal plane

flip angle 90°

transverse magnetisation

Fig. 1.19 Full longitudinal magnetisation is converted to full transverse magnetisation.

Pulse timing parameters

A very simplified pulse sequence is a combination of RF pulses, signals and intervening periods of recovery (Fig. 1.20). It is important to note that a pulse sequence as shown diagrammatically in Fig. 1.20 does not actually exist. It merely shows in simple terms the separate timing parameters used in more complicated sequences, i.e. TR and TE.

A pulse sequence consists of several components, the main ones are outlined below.

- The *repetition time (TR)* is the time from the application of one RF pulse to the application of the next RF pulse and is measured in milliseconds (ms). The TR determines the amount of relaxation that is allowed to occur between the end of one RF pulse and the application of the next. Therefore the TR determines the amount of T1 relaxation that has occurred.

- The *echo time (TE)* is the time from the application of the RF pulse to the peak of the signal induced in the coil and is also measured in ms. The TE determines how much decay of transverse magnetisation is allowed to occur before the signal is read. Therefore, the TE controls the amount of T2 relaxation that has occurred.

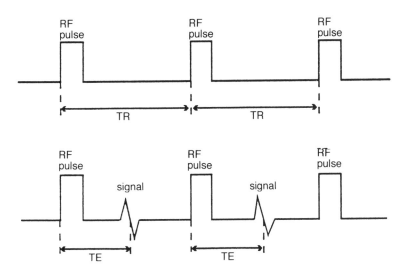

Fig. 1.20 A basic pulse sequence.

The basic principles of signal creation have now been described. The application of RF pulses at certain repetition times and the receiving of signals at pre-defined echo times produces contrast in MRI images. This concept is discussed fully in the next chapter.

Questions

1. What is the Larmor equation, and what does it calculate?

2. State the condition necessary for resonance to occur.

3. The energy difference between spin up and spin down nuclei depends on:
   (a) the Larmor frequency
   (b) the strength of the main magnetic field
   (c) the flip angle.

4. State the condition necessary for a signal to be generated in the receiver coil.

5. Define T1 recovery.

6. Define T2 decay.

7. Match the following relationships:

T1 recovery affects   the number of nuclei in the NMV

T2 decay affects   the angle of the NMV to the main magnetic field

Proton density affects   dephasing of magnetic moments in the NMV.

8. Do the TR or the TE determine the following?
   (a) Amount of T1 recovery.
   (b) Amount of T2 decay.

Chapter 2   Image Weighting and Contrast

Introduction

One of the main advantages of MRI compared with other imaging modalities is the excellent soft tissue discrimination of the images. The contrast characteristics of each image depend on many variables, and it is important that the mechanisms that affect image contrast in MRI are understood.

Image contrast

An image has contrast if there are areas of high signal (white on the image), as well as areas of low signal (dark on the image). Some areas have an intermediate signal (shades of grey in-between white and black). The NMV can be separated into the individual vectors of the tissues present in the patient such as fat, cerebrospinal fluid (CSF) and muscle.

A tissue has a high signal if it has a large transverse component of magnetisation. If there is a large component of transverse magnetisation the amplitude of the signal received by the coil is large resulting in a bright area on the image. A tissue returns a low signal, if it has a small transverse component of magnetisation. If there is a small component of transverse magnetisation the amplitude of the signal received by the coil is small resulting in a dark area on the image. Generally, the two extremes of contrast in MRI are *fat* and *water* (Fig. 2.1).

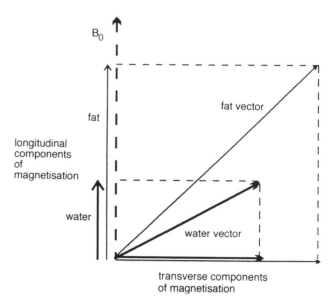

Fig. 2.1 Magnitude of transverse magnetisation versus amplitude of the signal. *Note* The frequencies of the signal are not representative in this diagram.

Fat and water

Fat is hydrogen linked to carbon and consists of large molecules called lipids. Water is hydrogen linked to oxygen which tends to steal the electrons away from around the hydrogen nucleus. This renders it more available to the effects of the main magnetic field. In fat, the carbon does not take the electrons from around the hydrogen nucleus. They remain in an electron cloud protecting the nucleus from the effects of the main field. Therefore the Larmor frequency of hydrogen in water is higher than hydrogen in fat. Hydrogen in fat recovers more rapidly along the longitudinal axis than water and loses transverse magnetisation faster than in water. Subsequently, fat and water appear differently in MR images.

Contrast mechanisms

Images obtain contrast mainly through the mechanisms of T1 recovery, T2 decay and proton or spin density. The proton density of a tissue is the number of protons per unit volume of that tissue.

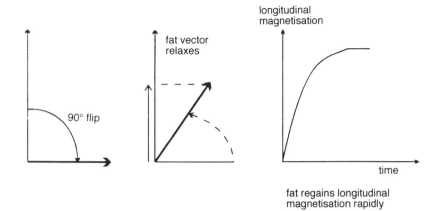

Fig. 2.2   T1 recovery in fat.

T1 recovery in fat

T1 recovery occurs due to nuclei giving up their energy to the surrounding environment. The slow molecular tumbling in fat allows the recovery process to be relatively rapid. This means that the magnetic moments of fat nuclei are able to relax and regain their longitudinal magnetisation quickly. The NMV of fat realigns rapidly with B_0 and therefore the T1 time of fat is short (Fig. 2.2).

T1 recovery in water

As we now know, T1 recovery occurs due to nuclei giving up the energy acquired from the RF excitation pulse to the surrounding lattice. In water,

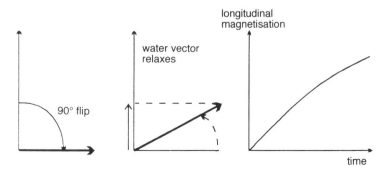

Fig. 2.3   T1 recovery in water.

molecular mobility is high resulting in less efficient T1 recovery. The magnetic moments of water take longer to relax and regain their longitudinal magnetisation. The NMV of water takes longer to realign with B_0 and so the T1 time of water is long (Fig. 2.3).

T2 decay in fat

T2 decay occurs as a result of the magnetic fields of the nuclei interacting with each other, thereby exchanging their energy to their neighbours. As energy exchange is more efficient in the hydrogen in fat, the T2 time is short. The T2 time of fat is approximately 80 ms (Fig. 2.4).

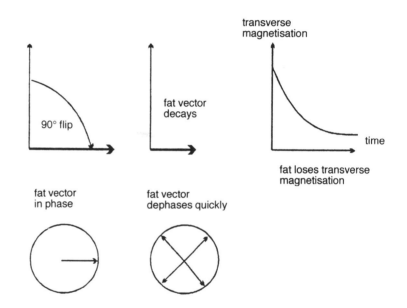

Fig. 2.4   T2 decay in fat.

T2 decay in water

As energy exchange in water is less efficient than in fat, the T2 time of hydrogen in water is long. The T2 time of water is approximately 200 ms (Fig. 2.5).

T1 contrast

As the T1 time of fat is shorter than water, the fat vector realigns with B_0 faster than that of water. The longitudinal component of magnetisation of fat is therefore larger than water. After a certain TR, the next RF excitation pulse is applied. The RF excitation pulse flips the longitudinal

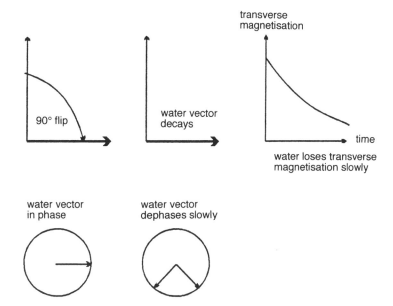

Fig. 2.5 T2 decay in water.

components of magnetisation of both fat and water into the transverse plane (assuming a 90° pulse is applied) as in Fig. 2.6.

As there is more longitudinal magnetisation in fat before the RF pulse, there is more transverse magnetisation in fat after the RF pulse. Fat therefore has a high signal and appears bright on a T1 contrast image. As there is less longitudinal magnetisation in water before the RF pulse, there is less transverse magnetisation in water after the RF pulse. Water therefore has a low signal and appears dark on a T1 contrast image. Such images are called T1 weighted images.

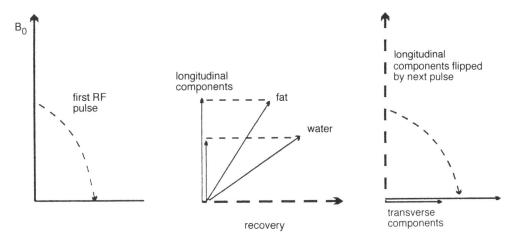

Fig. 2.6 T1 contrast.

T2 contrast

The T2 time of fat is shorter than that of water, therefore the transverse component of magnetisation of fat decays faster. The magnitude of transverse magnetisation in water is large. Water has a high signal and appears bright on a T2 contrast image. However, the magnitude of transverse magnetisation in fat is small. Fat therefore has a low signal, and appears dark on a T2 contrast image (Fig. 2.7). Such images are called T2 weighted images.

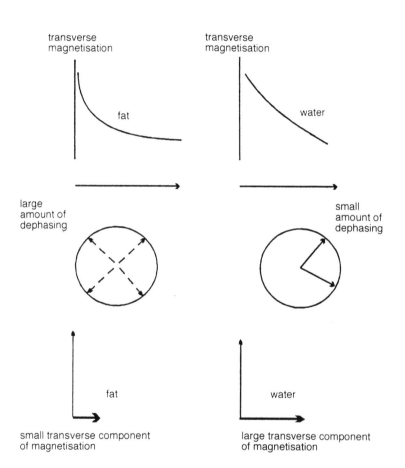

Fig. 2.7   T2 contrast.

Proton density contrast

Proton density contrast refers to differences in signal intensity between tissues which are a consequence of their relative number of protons per unit volume. To produce contrast due to the differences in the proton densities between the tissues, the transverse component of magnetisation must reflect these differences (Fig. 2.8). Tissues with a high proton density (e.g. brain tissue) have a large transverse component of magnetisation (and therefore a high signal), and are bright on a proton density contrast image. Tissues with a low proton density (e.g. cortical bone) have a small transverse component of magnetisation (and therefore a low signal), and are dark on a proton density contrast image. Proton density contrast is always present and depends on the patient and the area being examined. It is the basic MRI contrast.

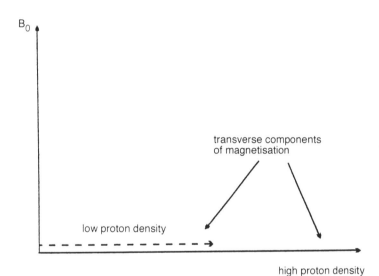

Fig. 2.8 Proton density contrast.

- Fat has a short T1 and T2 time.
- Water has a long T1 and T2 time.
- To produce high signal, there must be a large component of magnetisation in the transverse plane to induce a large signal in the coil.
- To produce a low signal, there must be a small component of magnetisation in the transverse plane to induce a small signal in the coil.
- T1 weighted images are characterised by bright fat and dark water.
- T2 weighted images are characterised by bright water and dark fat.
- Proton density weighted images are characterised by:
    areas with high proton density are bright,
    areas with low proton density are dark.

Weighting

To demonstrate either T1 proton density or T2 contrast, specific values of TR and TE are selected for a given pulse sequence. The selection of appropriate TR and TE weights an image so that one contrast mechanism predominates over the other two.

T1 weighting

A T1 weighted image is one where the contrast depends predominantly on the differences in the T1 times between fat and water (and therefore all the tissues with intermediate signal as well). Because the TR controls how far each vector can recover before it is excited by the next RF pulse, to achieve T1 weighting the TR must be short enough so that neither fat nor water has sufficient time to fully return to B_0. If the TR is too long, both fat and water return to B_0 and recover their longitudinal magnetisation fully. When this occurs, T1 relaxation is complete in both tissues and the differences in their T1 times are not demonstrated on the image (Fig. 2.9).

- TR controls the amount of T1 weighting.
- For T1 weighting the TR must be short.

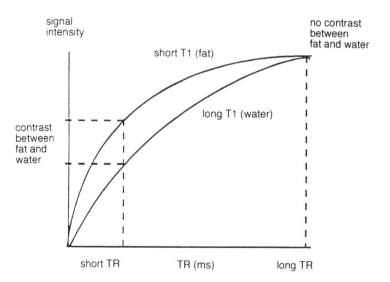

Fig. 2.9 The T1 differences between fat and water.

T2 weighting

A T2 weighted image is one where the contrast predominantly depends on the differences in the T2 times between fat and water (and therefore all the tissues with intermediate signal as well). The TE controls the amount of T2 decay that is allowed to occur before the signal is received. To achieve T2 weighting, the TE must be long enough to give both fat and water time to decay. If the TE is too short, neither fat nor water has had time to decay, and therefore the differences in their T2 times are not demonstrated in the image (Fig. 2.10).

- TE controls the amount of T2 weighting.
- For T2 weighting the TE must be long.

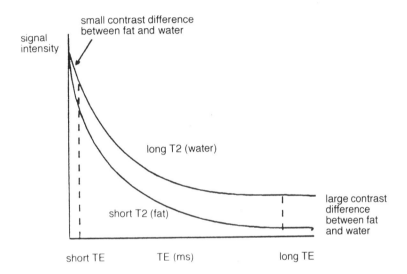

Fig. 2.10 T2 differences between fat and water.

Proton density weighting

A proton density image is one where the difference in the numbers of protons per unit volume in the patient is the main determining factor in forming image contrast. Proton density weighting is always present to some extent. In order to achieve proton density weighting, the effects of T1 and T2 contrast must be diminished, so that proton density weighting can dominate. A long TR allows both fat and water to fully recover their longitudinal magnetisation, and therefore diminishes T1 weighting. A short TE does not give fat or water time to decay and therefore diminishes T2 weighting.

In any image, the contrast due to the inherent proton density together with T1 and T2 mechanisms occur simultaneously and contribute to image contrast. In order to weight an image so that one process is dominant, the other processes must be diminished.

- For T1 weighting:
  - to exaggerate T1   TR is SHORT.
  - to diminish T2   TE is SHORT.
- For T2 weighting:
  - to exaggerate T2   TE is LONG.
  - to diminish T1   TR is LONG.
- For proton density weighting:
  - to diminish T2   TE is SHORT.
  - to diminish T1   TR is LONG.

LEARNING POINT

Whenever the NMV is pushed beyond 90° it is said to be *partially saturated*. When the NMV is pushed to a full 180° it is said to be *fully saturated*. If partial saturation of the fat and water vectors occurs T1 weighting results. If however saturation of the fat and water vectors does not occur, proton density weighting results. To understand this, the processes of T1 recovery should be reviewed.

Before the application of the first RF pulse, the fat and water vectors are aligned with B_0. When the first 90° RF pulse is applied, the fat and water vectors are flipped into the transverse plane. The RF pulse is then

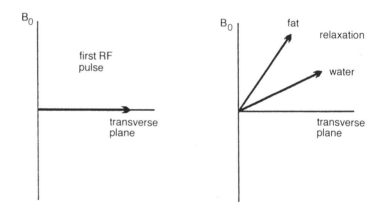

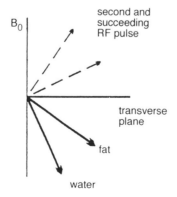

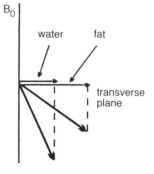

Fig. 2.11   Saturation.

removed, and the vectors begin to relax and return to B_0. Fat has a shorter T1 than water, and therefore returns to B_0 faster than water. If the TR is shorter than the T1 of the tissues, the next (and all succeeding) RF pulse, flips the vectors beyond 90° and into partial saturation because their recovery was incomplete. The fat and water vectors are saturated to different degrees because they were at different points of recovery before the 90° flip. The transverse component of magnetisation for each vector is therefore different. The transverse component of fat is greater than that of water because its longitudinal component grows to a greater degree before the next RF pulse is applied, and so more longitudinal magnetisation is available to be flipped into the transverse plane. The fat vector therefore generates a higher signal than water – fat is bright and water is dark. A T1 weighted image results (Fig. 2.11).

If the TR is longer than the T1 of the tissues, both fat and water fully recover before the next (and all succeeding) RF pulses are applied. Both vectors are flipped directly into the transverse plane and are never saturated. The magnitude of the transverse component of magnetisation for fat and water depends only on their individual proton densities, rather than the rate of recovery of their longitudinal components. Tissues with a high proton density are bright, whereas tissues with a low proton density are dark. A proton density weighted image results (Fig. 2.12).

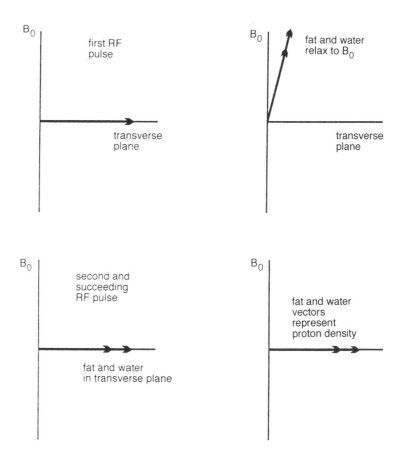

Fig. 2.12 No saturation.

Typical values of TR and TE

Long TR   2000 ms+
Short TR   250–700 ms
Long TE   60 ms+
Short TE   10–25 ms

T2* decay

When the RF excitation pulse is removed, the relaxation and decay processes occur immediately. T2* decay is the decay of the FID following the RF excitation pulse. This decay is faster than T2 decay since it is a combination of two effects, (1) T2 decay itself and (2) dephasing due to magnetic field inhomogeneities.

Inhomogeneities are areas within the magnetic field that do not exactly match the external magnetic field strength. Some areas have a magnetic field strength slightly less than the main magnetic field, whereas other areas have a magnetic field strength slightly more than the main magnetic field (Fig. 2.13).

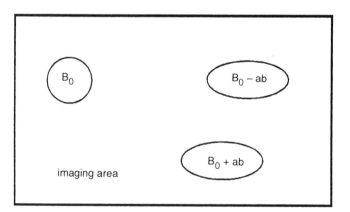

Fig. 2.13 Magnetic field inhomogeneities (ab represents these areas).

As the Larmor equation states, the Larmor frequency of a nucleus is proportional to the magnetic field strength it experiences. As a nucleus passes through an area of inhomogeneity with a higher field strength, the precessional frequency of the nucleus increases, i.e. it speeds up. However as a nucleus passes through an area of inhomogeneity with a lower field strength, the precessional frequency of the nucleus decreases, i.e. it slows down.

This relative acceleration and deceleration, as a result of magnetic field inhomogeneities and differences in the precessional frequency in certain tissues, causes immediate dephasing of the NMV (Fig. 2.14). This dephasing is predominantly responsible for T2* decay. The rate of dephasing due to inhomogeneities is an exponential process.

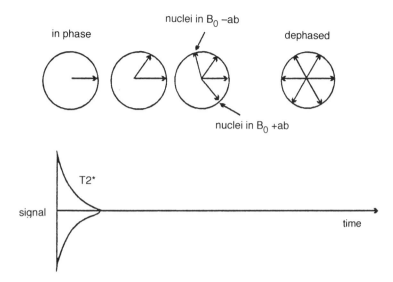

nuclei in B_0 $-ab$

in phase
dephased

nuclei in B_0 $+ab$

T2*

signal

time

Fig. 2.14 T2* decay.

Dephasing caused by inhomogeneities can be compensated for by a *180° RF pulse*. A pulse sequence that uses a 180° RF pulse to compensate for dephasing is called a *spin echo pulse sequence*.

The spin echo pulse sequence

The spin echo pulse sequence utilises a 90° excitation pulse to flip the NMV into the transverse plane. The NMV precesses in the transverse plane inducing a voltage in the receiver coil. The precessional paths of the magnetic moments of the nuclei within the NMV are translated into the

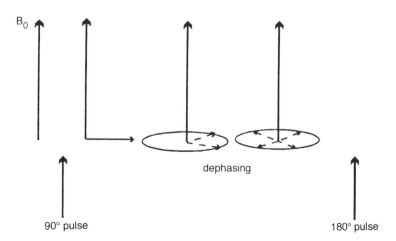

B_0

dephasing

Fig. 2.15 T2* dephasing.

90° pulse

180° pulse

transverse plane. When the 90° RF pulse is removed a free induction decay signal (FID) is produced. T2* dephasing occurs immediately, and the signal decays. A 180° RF pulse is then used to compensate for this dephasing (Fig. 2.15).

The 180° RF pulse is an RF pulse that has sufficient energy to move the NMV through 180°. The T2* dephasing causes the magnetic moments to dephase or 'fan out' in the transverse plane. The magnetic moments are now out of phase with each other, i.e. they are at different positions on the precessional path at any given time. The magnetic moments that slow down, form the trailing edge of the fan (S), and the magnetic moments that speed up, form the leading edge of the fan (F) (Fig. 2.16).

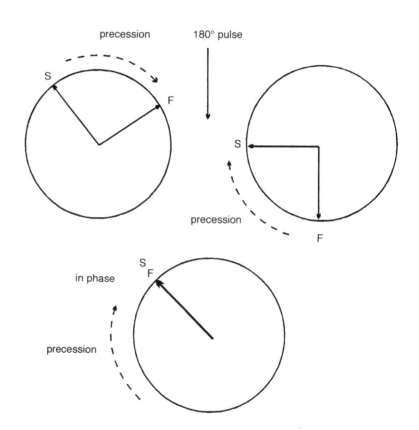

Fig. 2.16 180° rephasing.

The 180° RF pulse flips these individual magnetic moments through 180°. They are still in the transverse plane, but now the magnetic moments that formed the trailing edge before the 180° pulse, form the leading edge. Conversely, the magnetic moments that formed the leading edge prior to the 180° pulse, now form the trailing edge. The direction of precession remains the same, and so the trailing edge begins to catch up with the leading edge. At a specific time later, the two edges are superimposed. The magnetic moments are now momentarily in phase because they are momentarily at the same place on the precessional path. At this instant, there is transverse magnetisation in phase, and so a maximum signal is induced in the coil. This signal is called a *spin echo*. The spin echo now contains T1 and T2 information as T2* dephasing has been reduced (Fig. 2.17).

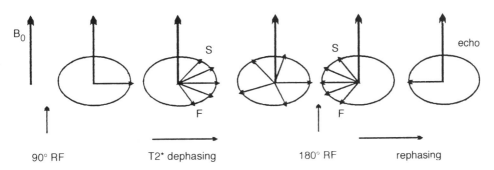

Fig. 2.17 RF rephasing

LEARNING POINT

An easy way to understand 180° rephasing is to use the analogy of the race track. Imagine three runners running around a circular race track. The runners relate to three magnetic moments and the circular race track to the precessional path of the magnetic moments. The runners have varying running ability; one is an Olympic runner (O), one a national runner (N), and one a very unfit amateur runner (A). At the sound of the start gun the runners set off around the track. Very shortly, the Olympic runner pulls ahead of the national runner, who in turn sprints ahead of the amateur. They are now out of phase with each other, as they are in a different place on the track to each other at a given time. The longer the race is allowed to run, the more dephasing between the runners occurs (Fig. 2.18).

The starting gun is fired again. The starting gun now refers to the 180° RF pulse. On hearing the gun, the runners turn around and head back towards the start line again. The Olympic runner is now at the back, because he ran further at the beginning of the race. The amateur runner is at the front because he ran slower at the beginning of the race. The national runner is somewhere in between. Assuming the runners run back to the start line at exactly the same speed as they ran at the beginning of the race, the Olympic and national runners catch up with the amateur, and are at exactly the same place at the same time when they get back to the start line (Fig. 2.19). They are therefore, back in phase, and if they were magnetic moments they would generate a spin echo at this point. The time taken for the runners to complete the whole race (from the starting line to the point where they turn around and back to the starting line again), corresponds to the TE.

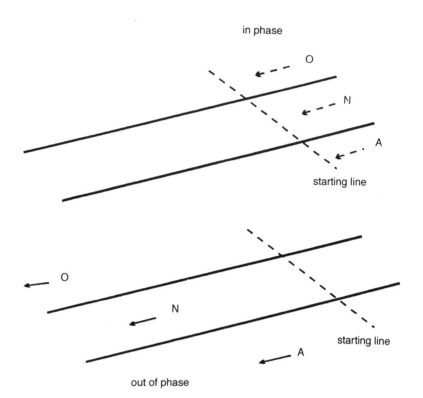

Fig. 2.18 The runners start the race.

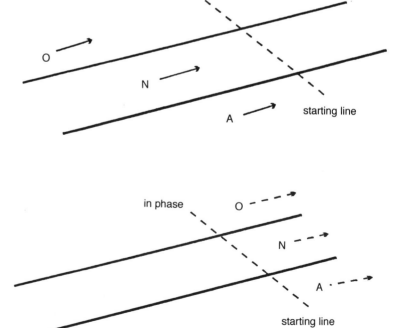

Fig. 2.19 The runners return.

Timing parameters in spin echo

TR is the time between each 90° excitation pulse. TE is the time between the 90° excitation pulse and the peak of the spin echo. The time taken to rephase after the application of the 180° RF pulse, equals the time the NMV took to dephase when the 90° RF pulse was withdrawn. This time is called the *TAU* time. The TE is therefore twice the TAU (Fig. 2.20).

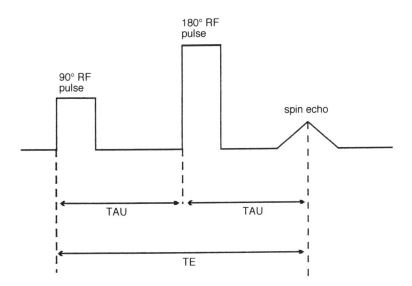

Fig. 2.20 The spin echo pulse sequence.

In most spin echo pulse sequences, more than one 180° RF pulse can be applied after the 90° excitation pulse. Each 180° pulse generates a separate spin echo that can be received by the coil and used to create an image. One, two or four 180° RF pulses can be used in spin echo, to produce either one, two or four images.

Spin echo using one echo

This pulse sequence can be used to produce T1 weighted images if a short TR and TE are used (Fig. 2.21). One 180° RF pulse is applied after the 90° excitation pulse. The single 180° RF pulse generates a single spin echo. The timing parameters used are selected to produce a T1 weighted image. A short TE ensures that the 180° RF pulse and subsequent echo occur early, so that only a little T2 decay has occurred. The differences in the T2 times of the tissues do not dominate the echo and its contrast. A short TR ensures that the fat and water vectors have not fully recovered, and so the differences in their T1 times dominate the echo and its contrast (Fig. 2.22).

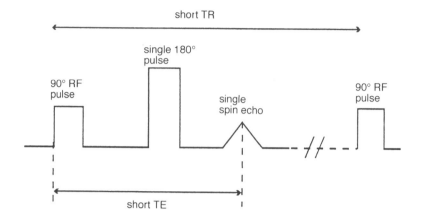

short TR

single 180°
pulse

90° RF
pulse

single
spin echo

90° RF
pulse

short TE

Fig. 2.21 What weighting do
you think this spin echo will
have?

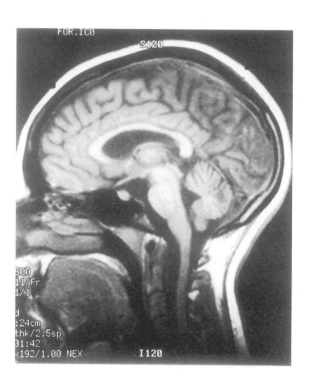

Fig. 2.22 T1 weighted sagittal
image of the brain, TE 11 ms,
TR 500 ms.

Spin echo using two echoes

This can be used to produce both a proton density and a T2 weighted
image in the TR time (Fig. 2.23). The first spin echo is generated early by
selecting a short TE. Only a little T2 decay has occurred and so T2
differences between the tissues are minimised in this echo. The second

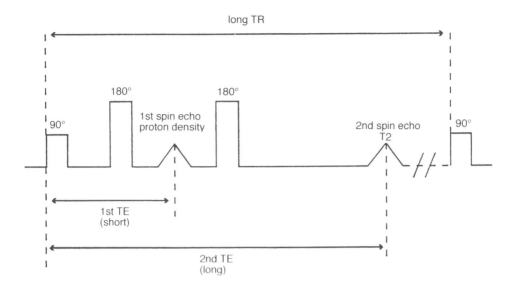

Fig. 2.23 A dual echo pulse sequence.

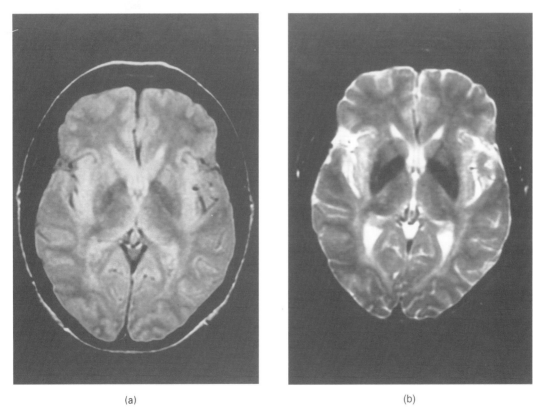

(a)　　　　　　　　　　　　　　　　(b)

Fig. 2.24(a) A proton density weighted axial image of the brain, TE 20 ms, TR 2700 ms. (b) A T2 weighted axial image of the brain, TE 90 ms, TR 2700 ms.

spin echo is generated much later by selecting a long TE. A significant amount of T2 decay has now occurred, and so the differences in the T2 times of the tissues are maximised in this echo. The TR selected is long, so that T1 differences between the tissues are minimised. The first spin echo therefore has a short TE and a long TR and is proton density weighted. The second spin echo has a long TE and a long TR and is T2 weighted. Figure 2.24 shows proton density and T2 weighted images.

- A spin echo pulse sequence uses a 90° excitation pulse followed by one or more 180° rephasing pulses to generate one or more spin echoes.
- Spin echo pulse sequences produce either T1, T2 or proton density weighting.
- TR controls the T1 weighting.
    Short TR maximises T1 weighting.
    Long TR maximises proton density weighting.
- TE controls the T2 weighting.
    Short TE minimises T2 weighting.
    Long TE maximises T2 weighting.

The gradient echo pulse sequence

A gradient echo pulse sequence utilises an RF excitation pulse that is variable, and therefore flips the NMV through any angle (not just 90°). A transverse component of magnetisation is created, the magnitude of which is less than in spin echo, where all the longitudinal magnetisation is converted to the transverse plane. When a flip angle other than 90° is used, only part of the longitudinal magnetisation is converted to transverse magnetisation, which precesses in the transverse plane and induces a signal in the receiver coil (Fig. 2.25).

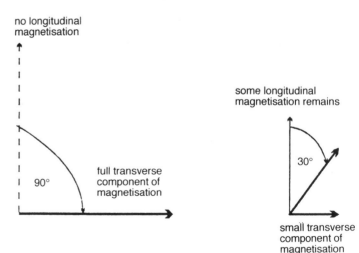

Fig. 2.25 How the flip angle controls the magnitude of the signal.

After the RF pulse is withdrawn, the FID signal is immediately produced due to inhomogeneities in the magnetic field and T2* dephasing therefore occurs. The magnetic moments within the transverse component of magnetisation dephase, and are then rephased by a *gradient*. A gradient causes a change in the magnetic field strength within the magnet and is discussed in more detail later. The gradient rephases the magnetic moments so that a signal can be received by the coil, which contains T1 and T2 information. This signal is called a *gradient echo*.

Gradients

Gradients perform many tasks that are explored fully in Chapter 3. Magnetic field gradients are generated by coils of wire situated within the bore of the magnet. The laws of electromagnetic induction state that when current is passed through a gradient coil, a magnetic field (or gradient field as it is now known) is induced around it. This gradient field interacts with the main static magnetic field, so that the magnetic field strength along the axis of the gradient coil is altered in a linear way. The middle of the axis of the gradient remains at the field strength of the main magnetic field. This is called *magnetic isocentre*. The magnetic field strength increases relative to isocentre in one direction of the gradient axis, and decreases

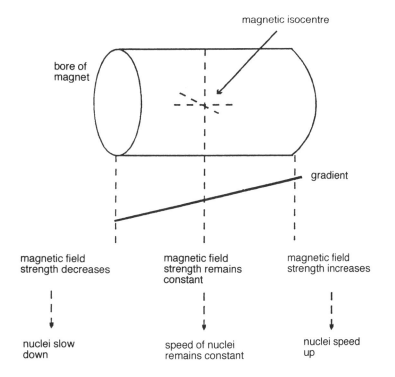

Fig. 2.26 The gradients.

relative to isocentre in the other direction of the gradient axis. The direction of the gradient that determines which end is high and which end is low is called the *polarity*. This is determined by the direction of the current in the gradient coil. When a gradient is switched on, the magnetic field strength along its axis is sloped or graded. The Larmor equation states that the precessional frequency of the magnetic moments increases or decreases, depending on the magnetic field strength they experience at different points along the gradient (Fig. 2.26). Therefore, the precessional frequency increases when the magnetic field increases and decreases when the magnetic field decreases.

- Magnetic moments experiencing an increased field strength due to the gradient speed up, i.e. their precessional frequency increases.
- Magnetic moments experiencing a decreased magnetic field strength slow down, i.e. their precessional frequency decreases.
- As gradients can cause nuclei to speed up or slow down, they can be used to either *dephase* or *rephase* their magnetic moments.

How gradients dephase

A gradient is applied to coherent (in phase) magnetisation (all the magnetic moments are in the same place at the same time). The gradient alters the magnetic field strength experienced by the coherent magnetisation. Depending on their position along the gradient axis some of the magnetic moments speed up and some slow down. Thus the magnetic moments fan out.

The trailing edge of the fan (S) consists of nuclei that have slowed down, as they are situated on the gradient axis that has a lower magnetic field strength relative to isocentre. The leading edge of the fan (F) consists of nuclei that have sped up as they are situated on the gradient axis that has a higher magnetic field strength relative to isocentre. The magnetic

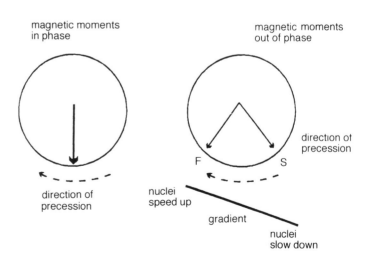

Fig. 2.27 How gradients dephase.

moments of the nuclei are therefore no longer in the same place at the same time and so the magnetisation has been dephased by the gradient (Fig. 2.27).

How gradients rephase

A gradient is applied to incoherent (out of phase) magnetisation. The magnetic moments have fanned out due to T2* dephasing and the fan has a trailing edge consisting of slow nuclei (S), and a leading edge consisting of faster nuclei (F). A gradient is then applied, so that the magnetic field strength is altered in a linear fashion along the axis of the gradient. The direction of this altered field strength is such that the slow nuclei in the trailing edge of the fan experience an increased magnetic field strength and speed up. The faster nuclei in the leading edge of the fan experience a decreased magnetic field strength and slow down. After a short period of time, the slow nuclei have sped up sufficiently to meet the faster nuclei that are slowing down (Fig. 2.28).

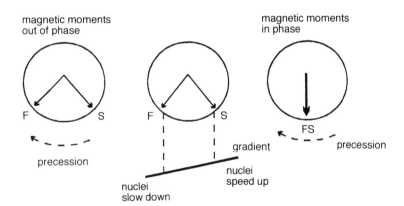

Fig. 2.28 How gradients rephase.

When the two meet, all the magnetic moments are in the same place at the same time and have been rephased by the gradient. A maximum signal is therefore induced in the receiver coil and this signal is called a *gradient echo*.

The advantages of gradient echo pulse sequences

Since gradients can rephase faster than 180° RF pulses the minimum TE is much shorter than in spin echo pulse sequences, and so the TR can also be reduced. The TR can also be reduced because flip angles other than 90° can be used. With low flip angles, full recovery of the longitudinal magnetisation occurs sooner than with large flip angles. The TR can therefore be shortened without producing saturation. The TR plays an important part in the time of the scan (see Chapter 3), so as the TR is reduced, the scan time is also reduced. Gradient echo pulse sequences are therefore usually associated with much shorter scan times than spin echo pulse sequences.

The disadvantages of gradient echo pulse sequences

The most important disadvantage is that there is no compensation for magnetic field inhomogeneities. Gradient echo pulse sequences are therefore very susceptible to magnetic field inhomogeneities. Gradient echo pulse sequences can contain magnetic susceptibility artefact (see Chapter 7). As the T2* effects are not eliminated, in gradient echo imaging T2 weighting is termed T2* weighting and T2 decay is termed T2* decay.

Timing parameters in gradient echo

As in spin echo, the TR is the time between each RF excitation pulse the TE is the time from the excitation pulse to the peak of gradient echo (Fig. 2.29).

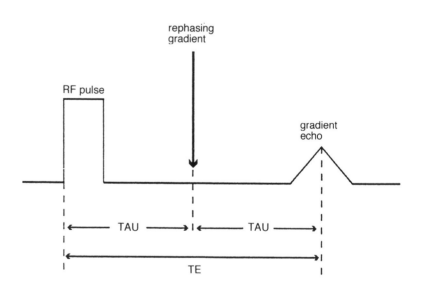

Fig. 2.29 The gradient echo pulse sequence.

Weighting and contrast in gradient echo

The TR, TE and flip angle affect image weighting and contrast and the TR can be much shorter than in spin echo pulse sequences. As the TR controls that amount of T1 recovery that has been allowed to occur before the application of the next RF pulse, a short TR produces T1 weighting and never permits a T2 or proton density weighted image to be obtained. To give gradient echo imaging more flexibility, the flip angle is reduced to less than 90°. If the flip angle is less than 90°, it does not take the NMV as long to recover full longitudinal magnetisation, and so the TR can be shortened to reduce the scan time without producing saturation (Fig. 2.30).

In gradient echo pulse sequences, the TR and the flip angle control the amount of T1 relaxation that has occurred before the next RF pulse is applied. The TE controls the amount of T2* decay that has occurred before the gradient echo is received by the coil. Apart from the added

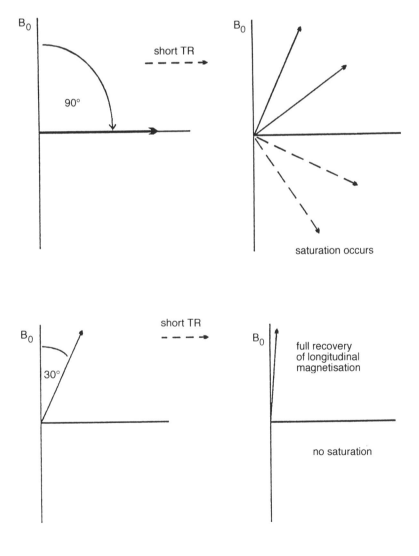

Fig. 2.30 How the TR and the flip angle control weighting.

variable of the flip angle, the rules of weighting in gradient echo are exactly the same as in spin echo.

T1 weighting in gradient echo

To obtain a T1 weighted image, the differences in the T1 times of the tissues are maximised, and the differences in the T2 times of the tissues are minimised. In order to maximise T1 differences, neither the fat nor water vectors must have had time to recover full longitudinal magnetisation before the next RF pulse is applied. To avoid full recovery, the flip angle is large and the TR short, so that the fat and water vectors are still in the process of relaxing when the next RF is applied. To minimise T2* differences, the TE is short so that neither fat nor water has had time to decay (Fig. 2.31).

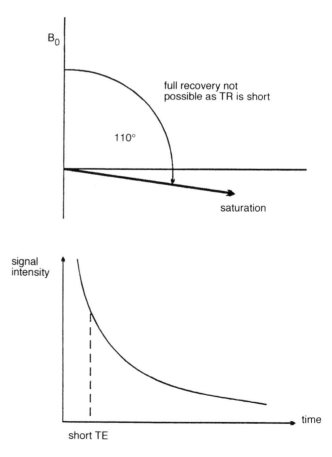

Fig. 2.31   T1 weighting in gradient echo.

T2* weighting in gradient echo

To obtain a T2* weighted image the differences in the T2* times of the tissues are maximised, and the differences in the T1 times are minimised. To maximise T2* decay, the TE is long so that the fat and water vectors have had time to decay sufficiently to show their decay differences. To minimise T1 recovery, the flip angle is small and the TR long enough to permit full recovery of the fat and water vectors. In this way, T1 differences are not demonstrated. In practice, small flip angles produce

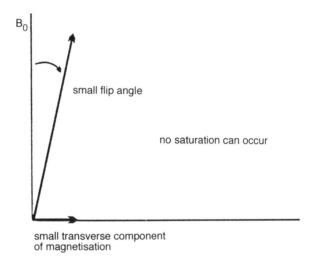

small flip angle

no saturation can occur

small transverse component
of magnetisation

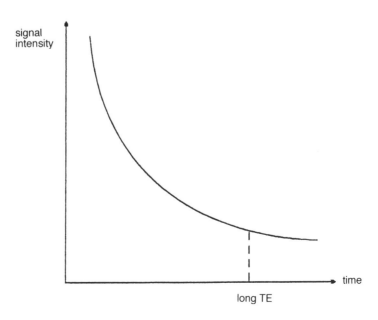

signal intensity

time

long TE

Fig. 2.32 T2* weighting in gradient echo.

such little transverse magnetisation, that the TR can be kept relatively short and full recovery still has time to occur (Fig. 2.32).

Proton density weighting in gradient echo

To obtain a proton density weighted image both T1 and T2* processes are minimised so that the differences in proton density of the tissues can be demonstrated. To minimise T2* decay, the TE is short so that neither the fat nor the water vectors have had time to decay. To minimise T1 recovery, the flip angle is small and the TR long enough to permit full recovery of longitudinal magnetisation.

- Gradient echo pulse sequences use a gradient to rephase the magnetic moments.
- Variable flip angles are used.
- The TE can be much shorter than in spin echo imaging.
- Gradients do not eliminate effects from magnetic field inhomogeneities.
- T1 weighting
  - to exaggerate T1   the flip angle is LARGE.
  - to exaggerate T1   TR is SHORT.
  - to diminish T2   TE is SHORT.
- T2* weighting
  - to diminish T1   the flip angle is SMALL.
  - to diminish T1   TR is fairly LONG (but in practice can still be short if the flip angle is small).
  - to exaggerate T2*   TE is LONG.
- Proton density weighting
  - to diminish T1   the flip angle is SMALL.
  - to diminish T1   TR is fairly LONG.
  - to diminish T2*   TE is SHORT.

Typical values in gradient echo imaging

Long TR	100 ms+
Short TR	less than 50 ms
Short TE	5–10 ms
Long TE	15–25 ms
Low flip angles	5°–20°
Large flip angles	70°–110°

Table 2.1 summarises the differences between spin echo and gradient echo. Table 2.2 gives the parameters used in gradient echo. Signal creation and how it can be manipulated to produce image contrast has now been discussed. In the next chapter, the process of image formation is described.

Table 2.1 Summary of the differences between spin echo and gradient echo.

	TR	TE	Flip angle
Spin echo	long 2000 ms+	long 60 ms+	90° (usually)
	short 250–700 ms	short 10–25 ms	90° (usually)
Gradient echo	long 100 ms+	long 15–25 ms	small 5°–20°
			large 70°–110°
	short less than 50 ms	short 5–10 ms	small 5°–20°
			large 70°–110°

Table 2.2 Parameters used in gradient echo.

	TR	TE	Flip angle
T1 weighting	short	short	large
T2* weighting	fairly long	long	small
Proton density weighting	fairly long	short	small

Questions

1. Define the term *weighting*.

2. What is meant by:
   (a) a T1 weighted image?
   (b) a T2 weighted image?
   (c) a proton density weighted image?

3. When saturation occurs:
   (a) the NMV is pushed beyond the transverse plane
   (b) the magnetic moments dephase
   (c) the MR signal is received.

4. What values of TR and TE are needed for T1 weighting and why?

5. Why do we use a 180° RF pulse in spin echo?

6. List three main factors that make gradient echo sequences different from spin echo.

7. What parameters control T1 and proton density weighting in gradient echo?

8. What type of contrast will the following produce?
   (a) TR 400 ms, TE 5 ms, flip 120°.
   (b) TR 50 ms, TE 15 ms, flip 35°.

Chapter 3   Encoding and Image Formation

ENCODING

Introduction

As previously described, for resonance to occur RF must be applied at 90° to B_0 at the precessional frequency of hydrogen. This RF gives the NMV energy so that it is flipped into the transverse plane. The RF pulse also puts the individual magnetic moments that constitute the NMV into phase. The resultant coherent transverse magnetisation precesses at the Larmor frequency of hydrogen in the transverse plane. A voltage or signal is therefore induced in the receiver coil that is positioned in the transverse plane. This signal has a frequency equal to the Larmor frequency of hydrogen, regardless of the origin of the signal in the patient. For example:

at 1.5 T the frequency of hydrogen is 63.86 MHz,
at 1.0 T the frequency of hydrogen is 42.57 MHz,
at 0.5 T the frequency of hydrogen is 21.28 MHz.

The system must be able to locate the signal spatially in three dimensions, so that it can position each signal at the correct point on the image. First it locates a slice. Once a slice is selected, the signal is located or encoded along both axes of the image. These tasks are performed by gradients.

Gradients

Gradients are alterations to the main magnetic field and are generated by coils of wire located within the bore of the magnet through which current is passed. The passage of current through a gradient coil induces a gradient (magnetic) field around it, that either subtracts from, or adds to, the main static magnetic field strength B_0. The magnitude of B_0 is altered in a linear fashion by the gradient coils, so that the magnetic field strength and therefore the precessional frequency experienced by nuclei situated along the axis of the gradient can be predicted (Fig. 3.1). This is called spatial encoding.

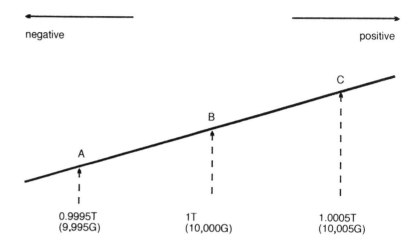

Fig. 3.1 What do you think the precessional frequency will be at A, B, and C, if the field strength is 0.5 T and 1.5 T?

Nuclei that experience an increased magnetic field strength due to the gradient speed up, i.e. their precessional frequency increases; whereas nuclei that experience a lower magnetic field strength due to the gradient slow down, i.e. their precessional frequency decreases. Therefore the position of a nucleus along a gradient can be identified according to its precessional frequency. Table 3.1 gives the frequency changes along a linear gradient that alters the magnetic field strength by 1 G/cm.

Table 3.1 Frequency changes along a linear gradient.

Position along gradient	Field strength	Larmor frequency
at isocentre	10 000 G	42.5700 MHz
1 cm negative to isocentre	9 999 G	42.5657 MHz
2 cm negative to isocentre	9 998 G	42.5614 MHz
1 cm positive to isocentre	10 001 G	42.5742 MHz
2 cm positive to isocentre	10 002 G	42.5785 MHz
10 cm negative to isocentre	9 990 G	42.5274 MHz

There are three gradient coils situated within the bore of the magnet, and these are named according to the axis along which they act when they are switched on (Fig. 3.2).

- The *Z gradient* alters the magnetic field strength along the Z- *(long) axis* of the magnet
- The *Y gradient* alters the magnetic field strength along the Y- *(vertical) axis* of the magnet
- The *X gradient* alters the magnetic field strength along the X- *(horizontal) axis* of the magnet
- The *magnetic isocentre* is the centre point of the axis of all three gradients, and the bore of the magnet. The magnetic field strength remains unaltered here even when the gradients are applied.

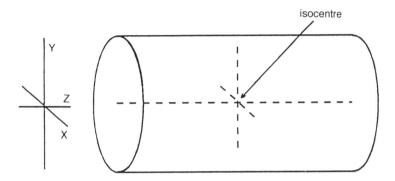

Fig. 3.2 The X, Y and Z gradient axes.

Table 3.2 Gradient axes in orthogonal plane imaging.

	Slice selection	Phase encoding	Frequency encoding
Sagittal	X	Y	Z
Axial (body)	Z	Y	X
Axial (head)	Z	X	Y
Coronal	Y	X	Z

The magnetic field strength at the isocentre is always the same as B_0 (1.5 T, 1.0 T, 0.5 T), even when the gradients are switched on. When a gradient coil is switched on, the magnetic field strength is either subtracted from or added to B_0 relative to isocentre. The slope of the resulting magnetic field is the amplitude of the magnetic field gradient and it determines the rate of change of the magnetic field strength along the gradient axis. Steep gradient slopes alter the magnetic field strength between two points more than shallow gradient slopes. Steep gradient slopes therefore alter the precessional frequency of nuclei between two points, more than shallow gradient slopes (Fig. 3.3).

It is convenient (for easy mathematics) to now use the unit gauss to describe magnetic field strength rather than tesla.

1.0 T is equal to 10 000 G

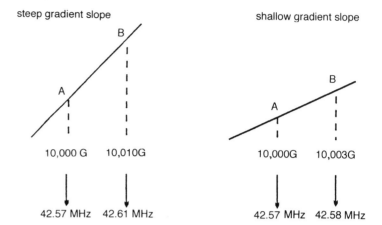

Fig. 3.3 Steep and shallow gradient slopes.

Gradients perform many important tasks during a pulse sequence. As previously described, gradients can be used to either dephase or rephase the magnetic moments of nuclei. Gradients also perform the following three main tasks in encoding.

(1) Slice selection – locating a slice within the scan plane selected.
(2) Spatially locating (encoding) signal along the long axis of the anatomy – this is called *frequency encoding*.
(3) Spatially locating (encoding) signal along the short axis of the anatomy – this is called *phase encoding*.

Slice selection

When a gradient coil is switched on, the magnetic field strength, and therefore the precessional frequency of nuclei located along its axis, are altered in a linear fashion. Therefore a specific point along the axis of the gradient has a specific precessional frequency. A slice situated at a certain point along the axis of the gradient has a particular precessional frequency. A slice can therefore be selectively excited, by transmitting RF with a band of frequencies coinciding with the Larmor frequencies of spins in a particular slice as defined by the slice select gradient. Resonance of nuclei within the slice occurs because RF appropriate to that position is transmitted. However, nuclei situated in other slices along the gradient do not resonate, because their precessional frequency is different due to the presence of the gradient (Fig. 3.4).

A specific slice is therefore excited and located within the patient. The scan plane selected determines which of the three gradients performs slice selection during the pulse sequence (Fig. 3.5).

● The *Z gradient* alters the field strength and precessional frequency along the Z axis of the magnet and therefore selects *axial slices*.

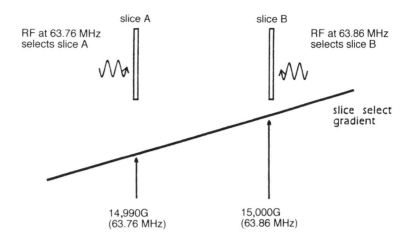

Fig. 3.4 Slice selection.

- The X *gradient* alters the field strength and the precessional frequency along the X axis of the magnet and therefore selects *sagittal slices*.
- The Y *gradient* alters the field strength and the precessional frequency along the Y axis of the magnet and therefore selects *coronal slices*.
- Oblique slices are selected using two gradients in combination.

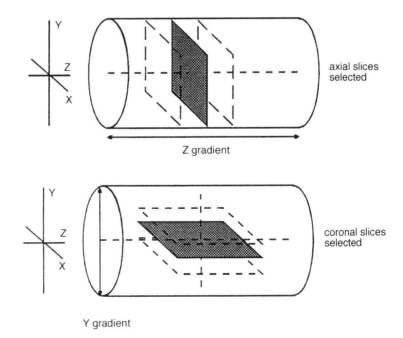

Fig. 3.5 The Y and Z gradients as slice selectors.

Slice thickness

To give each slice a thickness, a 'band' of nuclei must be excited by the excitation pulse. The slope of the slice-select gradient determines the difference in precessional frequency between two points on the gradient.

Steep gradient slopes result in a large difference in precessional frequency between two points on the gradient, whereas shallow gradient slopes result in a small difference in precessional frequency between the same two points. Once a certain gradient slope is applied, the RF pulse transmitted to excite the slice, must contain a range of frequencies to match the difference in precessional frequency between two points. This frequency range is called the *bandwidth*, and as the RF is being transmitted at this point it is specifically called the *transmit bandwidth* (Fig. 3.6).

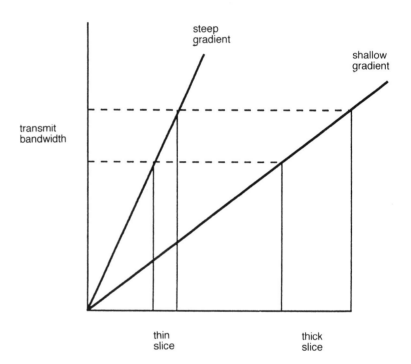

Fig. 3.6 Transmit bandwidth and gradient slope versus slice thickness.

- To achieve *thin slices*, a *steep* slice select slope and/or *narrow bandwidth* is applied.
- To achieve *thick slices*, a *shallow* slice select slope and/or *broad transmit bandwidth* is applied.

In practice, the system automatically applies the appropriate gradient slope and transmit bandwidth according to the thickness of slice required. The slice is excited by transmitting RF at the centre frequency corresponding to the precessional frequency of nuclei in the middle of the slice, and the bandwidth and gradient slope determine the range of nuclei that resonate on either side of the centre.

The gap between the slices is determined by the gradient slope and by the thickness of the slice. The size of the gap is important in reducing image artefact (see Chapter 7). In spin echo pulse sequences, the slice select gradient is switched on during the application of the 90° excitation pulse and during the 180° rephasing pulse, to excite and rephase each slice selectively (Fig. 3.7). In gradient echo pulse sequences, the slice-select gradient is switched on during the excitation pulse only. The significance of this is explored in Chapter 6.

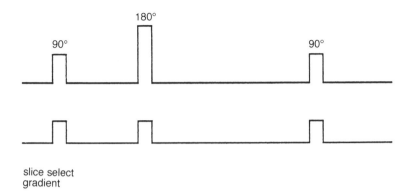

Fig. 3.7 The timing of slice selection in spin echo.

slice select gradient

Frequency encoding

Once a slice has been selected, the signal coming from it must be located along both axes of the image. The signal is usually located along the long axis of the anatomy by a process known as frequency encoding. When the frequency encoding gradient is switched on, the magnetic field strength and therefore the precessional frequency of signal along the axis of the gradient, is altered in a linear fashion. The gradient therefore produces a frequency difference or shift of signal along its axis. The signal can now be located along the axis of the gradient according to its frequency (Fig. 3.8).

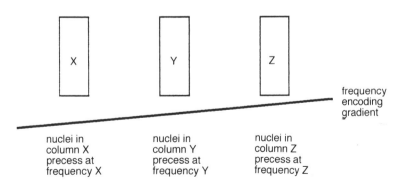

Fig. 3.8 Frequency shift.

The direction of frequency encoding can be selected by the operator so that it encodes the signal along the long axis of the anatomy.

- In *coronal* and *sagittal images*, the long axis of the anatomy lies along the Z axis of the magnet and therefore, the *Z gradient* performs frequency encoding.

- In *axial images*, the long axis of the anatomy usually lies along the horizontal axis of the magnet and therefore, the X *gradient* performs frequency encoding. However in imaging of the head, the long axis of the anatomy usually lies along the anterior posterior axis of the magnet, so in this case, the Y gradient will perform frequency encoding.

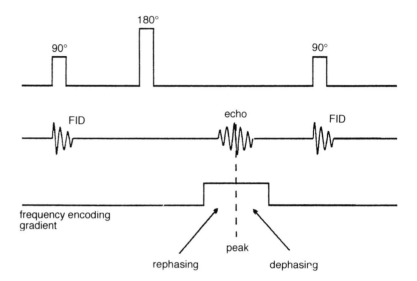

Fig. 3.9 The timing of frequency encoding in spin echo.

The frequency encoding gradient is switched on when the signal is received and is often called the *readout gradient*. The echo is usually centred in the middle of the frequency encoding gradient, so that the gradient is switched on during the rephasing and dephasing part of the echo as well as the peak (Fig. 3.9). For example, the frequency encoding gradient is switched on for 8 ms, and during 4 ms of rephasing and 4 ms of dephasing. The steepness of the slope of the frequency encoding gradient determines the size of the anatomy covered along the frequency encoding axis during the scan. This is called the *field of view (FOV)*.

Phase encoding

Signal must now be located along the remaining axis of the image and this localisation of signal is called phase encoding. When the phase encoding gradient is switched on, the magnetic field strength and therefore the precessional frequency of nuclei along the axis of the gradient is altered. As the speed of precession of the nuclei changes, so does the accumulated phase of the magnetic moments along their precessional path. Nuclei that have sped up due to the presence of the gradient, move further around their precessional path than if the gradient had not been applied. Nuclei that have slowed down due to the presence of the gradient, move further back around their precessional path than if the gradient had not been applied (Fig. 3.10).

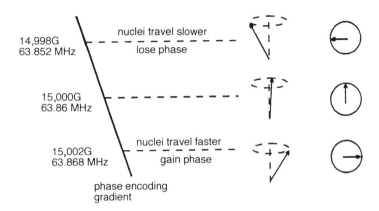

Fig. 3.10 Phase shift.

LEARNING POINT

It may help to compare the phase of magnetic moments around their precessional paths with the hands on a clock (Fig. 3.11). If the circular precessional path of the magnetic moments is turned vertically, the position of the magnetic moments on the face of the clock relates to their phase at a certain time. When the phase encoding gradient is switched off, all the nuclei precess at the Larmor frequency and have a phase of say, 12 o'clock. When the phase encoding gradient is switched on, the magnetic field strength, precessional frequency, and phase of the nuclei change according to their position along the gradient. Nuclei experiencing a higher field strength gain phase, i.e. move further around the clock to say 3 o'clock, whereas nuclei experiencing a lower field strength lose phase, i.e. move back around the clock to say 9 o'clock. Nuclei at the isocentre do not experience a changed field strength and their phase remains unchanged, i.e. 12 o'clock.

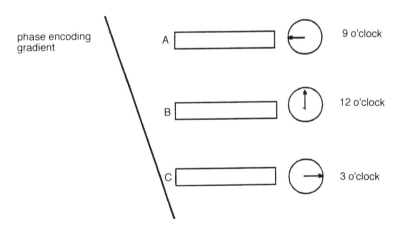

Fig. 3.11 Think of phase as the hands of a clock.

There is now a phase difference or shift between nuclei positioned along the axis of the gradient. When the phase encoding gradient is switched off, the magnetic field strength experienced by the nuclei returns to the main field strength B_0, and therefore the precessional frequency of all the nuclei returns to the Larmor frequency. However, the phase difference between the nuclei remains. The nuclei travel at the same speed around their precessional paths, but their phases or positions on the clock, are different. This difference in phase between the nuclei is used to determine their position along the phase encoding gradient.

The phase encoding gradient is usually switched on just before the application of the 180° rephasing pulse. The steepness of the slope of the phase encoding gradient determines the degree of phase shift between two points along the gradient (Fig. 3.12).

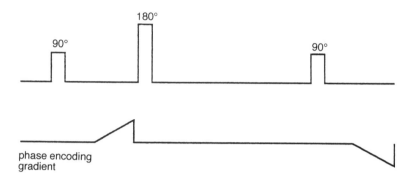

Fig. 3.12 The timing of phase encoding in spin echo.

A steep phase encoding gradient causes a large phase shift between two points along the gradient, for example 12 o'clock and 6 o'clock, whereas a shallow phase encoding gradient causes a smaller phase shift between two points along the gradient, for example 12 o'clock and 3 o'clock (Fig. 3.13).

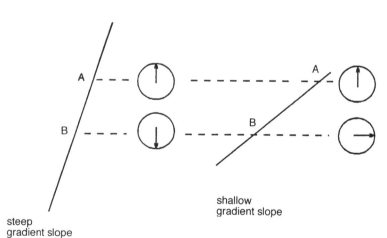

Fig. 3.13 The relationship between phase encoding gradient slope and phase shift.

Figure 3.14, Table 3.2 and the following list summarise the essential concepts of spatial encoding.

- The phase encoding gradient alters the phase along the remaining axis of the image, which is usually the short axis of the anatomy.
- In *coronal images* the short axis of the anatomy usually lies along the horizontal axis of the magnet, and therefore, the *X gradient* performs phase encoding.

- In *sagittal images* the short axis of the anatomy usually lies along the vertical axis of the magnet and therefore the Y *gradient* performs phase encoding.
- In *axial images*, the short axis of the anatomy usually lies along the vertical axis of the magnet, and therefore, the Y *gradient* performs phase encoding. However, when imaging the head, the short axis of the anatomy lies along the horizontal axis of the magnet and therefore the X gradient performs phase encoding.
- The slice-select gradient is switched on during the 90 and 180° pulses in spin echo pulse sequences, and during the excitation pulse only in gradient echo pulse sequences.
- The slope of the slice-select gradient determines the slice thickness and slice gap (along with the transmit bandwidth).
- The phase encoding gradient is switched on just before the 180° pulse in spin echo, and between excitation and the signal collection in gradient echo.
- The slope of the phase encoding gradient determines the degree of phase shift along the phase encoding axis.
- The frequency encoding gradient is switched on during the collection of the signal.
- The amplitude of the frequency encoding gradient and the phase encoding gradient determines the two dimensions of the FOV.

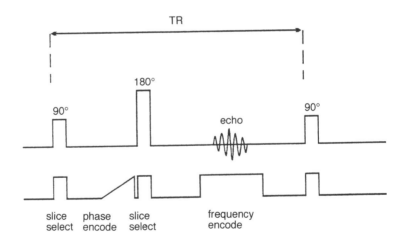

Fig. 3.14 Gradient timing in spin echo.

Sampling

The frequency encoding gradient is switched on during the collection of the signal, and is therefore, often called the readout gradient. The duration of the frequency encoding gradient during readout is called the *sampling time*. During the sampling time the system samples up to 1024 different frequencies (using current technology). The *sampling rate* is the rate at which the samples are taken during readout. The number of samples taken determines the number of frequencies that are sampled. During the sampling time, the system must be able to receive and sample a range of frequencies, and as signal is being received at this point, this range of frequencies is called the *receive bandwidth*. Each frequency is allocated a frequency column that is mapped onto the FOV along the frequency axis (Fig. 3.15).

frequency columns
in FOV

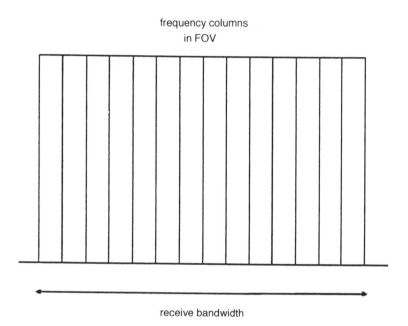

Fig. 3.15 Frequencies sampled are mapped across the FOV.

receive bandwidth

The sampling time, sampling rate and receive bandwidth are all linked by a mathematical principle called the *Nyquist theorem*. The Nyquist theorem states that any signal must be sampled at least twice per cycle in order to represent, or reproduce it accurately (Fig. 3.16). In addition, enough cycles must occur during the sampling time to achieve enough frequency samples. For example, if 256 samples are to be taken, at least 128 cycles must occur during the sampling time if each cycle is sampled twice.

The number of cycles occurring per second is determined by the receive bandwidth which is proportional to the sampling rate, i.e. if the sampling rate increases, the bandwidth also increases. In addition, the sampling time is inversely proportional to the sampling rate and to the receive bandwidth, so if the receive bandwidth is reduced, the sampling time increases.

- Sampling *rate* is proportional to the receive bandwidth.
- Sampling *time* is inversely proportional to:
  (1) the sampling rate,
  (2) the receive bandwidth.

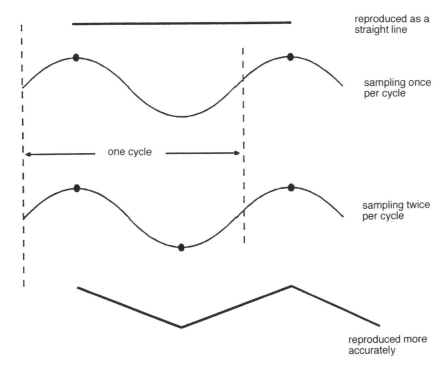

Fig. 3.16 The Nyquist theorem.

LEARNING POINT

To understand sampling more clearly, assume a receive bandwidth of 16 000 Hz and a sampling time of 8 ms. 16 000 cycles therefore occur per second, so that 128 cycles occur during the sampling time (8 ms). If 256

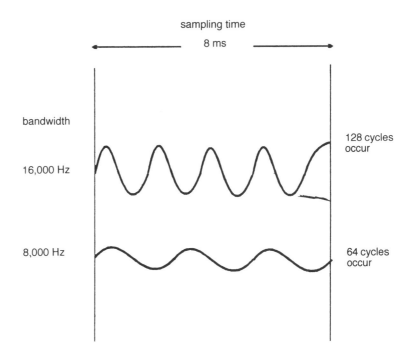

Fig. 3.17 Bandwidth versus the sampling time.

LEARNING POINT

continued

frequency samples are to be taken during this 8 ms and each cycle is sampled twice (Nyquist theorem), each of the 128 cycles can be sampled twice to obtain the 256 samples required. However if the bandwidth is reduced to say 8000 Hz, only 64 cycles occur in 8 ms. If the Nyquist theorem is to be obeyed, only 128 samples can be taken from these 64 cycles (which is not enough, as 256 samples are required). In other words, 128 cycles must occur during the sampling time in order to sample each cycle twice and obtain the 256 samples. Therefore if the bandwidth is reduced, the sampling time must increase so that 128 cycles can occur and 256 samples can be taken (Fig. 3.17).

Reducing the receive bandwidth affects the minimum TE because the echo is usually centred on the middle of the frequency encoding gradient. Increasing the sampling time means that the frequency encoding gradient is switched on for longer and therefore the position of the centre of the echo moves further away from the RF excitation pulse, i.e. the TE is increased (Fig. 3.18).

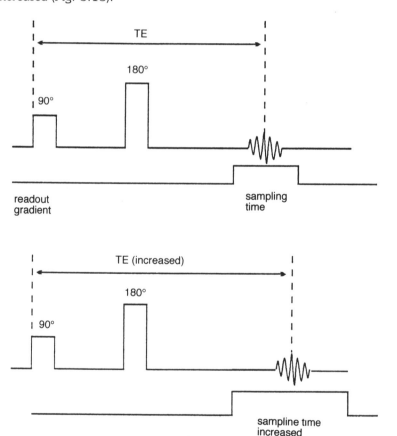

Fig. 3.18 The sampling time and the TE.

Under normal circumstances the receive bandwidth and sampling time are fixed, for example the receive bandwidth is $\pm 16\,000$ Hz and the sampling time is 8 ms. However, there are occasions when it is desirable to alter the receive bandwidth and this is when the increase in TE may become significant. These considerations are discussed later. Since signal encoding has been explored, the process of mapping the encoded signal into the FOV is now discussed.

DATA COLLECTION AND IMAGE FORMATION

Introduction

The application of all the gradients selects an individual slice and produces a frequency shift along one axis of the slice, and a phase shift along the other. The system can now locate an individual signal within the image by measuring the number of times the magnetic moments cross the receiver coil, (frequency) and their position around their precessional path (phase) (Fig. 3.19). This information now has to be translated on to the image. When data of each signal position is collected, the information is stored in the array processor of the system computer. The data information is stored in *K space*.

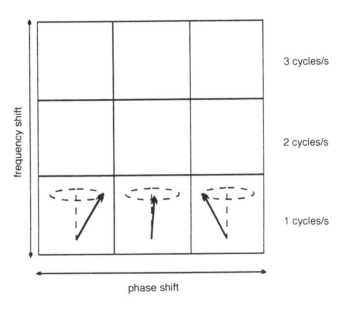

Fig. 3.19 Phase and frequency shift.

K space

K space is rectangular in shape and has two axes perpendicular to each other. The phase axis of K space is horizontal and is centred in the middle of several horizontal lines. The frequency axis of K space is vertical and is centred in the middle of K space perpendicular to the phase axis (Fig. 3.20). K space is a spatial frequency domain, i.e. where information about the frequency of a signal and where it comes from in the patient is stored. As frequency is defined as phase change per unit time and is measured in radians, the unit of K space is radians per cm.

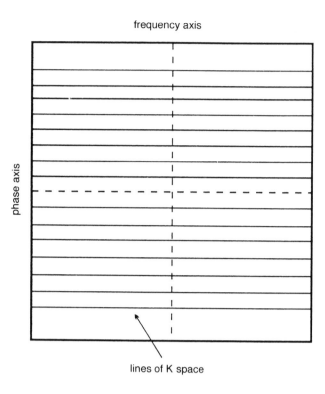

frequency axis

phase axis

Fig. 3.20 K space.

lines of K space

K space is analogous to the lens of a camera. When using a camera to photograph an object, light passes from the object through the lens of the camera and onto a film. The lens processes the light it receives from the object so that it forms a latent image of the object on the film. In MR the object is a patient and in order to produce an image, RF from the patient is stored in K space and later processed. In fact both an optical lens and K space use Fourier mathematics to produce images – the lens uses light energy whereas K space uses RF energy. Every time a frequency or phase encoding is performed, data is collected and stored in one of the lines of K space. This data is later processed to produce an image of the patient. It is very important to understand that K space does not correspond to the image, i.e. the top line of K space does not correspond with the top line of the image. K space is merely an area where data is stored until the scan is over.

Data collection – Step 1

During each TR, the signal from each slice is phase encoded and frequency encoded. A certain value of frequency shift is obtained according to the slope of the frequency encoding gradient which is, in turn, determined by the size of the FOV. As the FOV remains unchanged during the scan, the frequency shift value remains the same. A certain value of phase shift is also obtained according to the slope of the phase encoding gradient. The slope of the phase encoding gradient, will determine which line of K space is filled with the data from that frequency and phase encoding. In order to fill out different lines of K space, the slope of the phase encoding gradient must be altered after each TR. If the slope of the phase encoding gradient is not altered, the same line of K space is filled in all the time. In order to finish the scan or *acquisition*, all the selected lines of K space must be filled. The number of lines of K space that are filled, is determined by the number of different phase encoding slopes that are applied (Fig. 3.21).

- If 128 different phase encoding slopes are selected, 128 lines of K space are filled to complete the scan.
- If 256 different phase encoding slopes are selected, 256 lines of K space are filled to complete the scan.

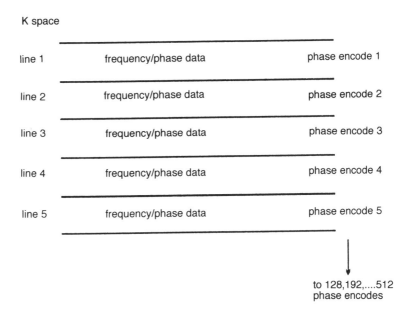

K space

line 1	frequency/phase data	phase encode 1
line 2	frequency/phase data	phase encode 2
line 3	frequency/phase data	phase encode 3
line 4	frequency/phase data	phase encode 4
line 5	frequency/phase data	phase encode 5

to 128,192,....512
phase encodes

Fig. 3.21   K space lines.

The slope of the phase encoding gradient determines the magnitude of the phase shift between two points in the patient. Steep slopes produce a large phase difference between two points, whereas shallow slopes produce small phase shifts between the same two points. The system cannot however measure phase directly, it can only measure frequency. The system therefore converts the phase shift into a frequency.

As frequency is a change of phase over time, phase shift values are converted into frequencies by creating a sine wave formed from connecting all the phase values associated with a certain phase shift (see Fig. 3.22). This sine wave has a certain frequency or *pseudo-frequency* (as it has been indirectly obtained). After all the phase encoding steps have been acquired and stored in K space, the phase shift values are converted into pseudo-frequencies.

In order to fill a different line of K space, a different phase shift must be

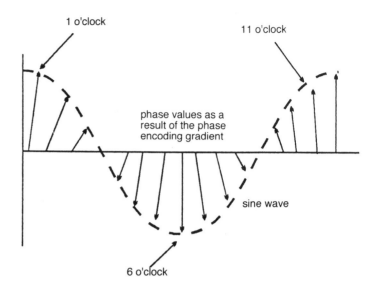

Fig. 3.22 The sine wave.

obtained. If a different phase shift is not obtained, the same line of K space is filled over and over again. To create a different phase shift the phase encoding gradient is switched on to a different amplitude or slope. Therefore, the change in phase shift created by the altered phase encoding gradient slope results in a sine wave with a different pseudo-frequency (Fig. 3.23).

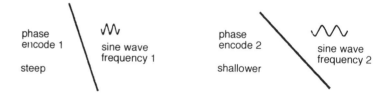

Fig. 3.23 Phase encoding slope versus pseudo-frequency.

- Every TR, each slice is frequency encoded (resulting in the same frequency shift), and phase encoded with a different slope of phase encoding gradient to produce a different pseudo-frequency.
- Usually different lines in K space are filled after every TR.
- Once all the lines of selected K space have been filled, the acquisition of data is complete and the scan is over.

The acquired data held in K space is now converted into an image. This conversion is made mathematically by a process known as *Fast Fourier Transform (FFT)*.

Fast Fourier Transform (FFT)

It is well beyond the scope of this book to study the intricacies of FFT. Suffice it to say that it is purely a mathematical process. The FID is initially measured as a relationship of its frequency against time. The FFT process mathematically converts this to calculate the amplitude of individual frequencies. The signal intensity/time domain is therefore converted to a signal intensity/frequency domain. As the FFT process deals in frequencies, the system must acquire both phase and frequency shifts in frequencies (Fig. 3.24). This is why it is necessary to convert the phase shift produced as a result of the application of each of the phase gradients into a frequency.

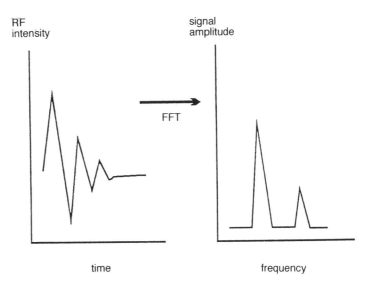

Fig. 3.24 The Fast Fourier Transform.

Matrix

The image consists of a FOV that relates to the amount of anatomy covered. The FOV can be square or rectangular, and is divided up into pixels or picture elements. The number of pixels within the FOV depends on the number of frequency samples and phase encodings performed. The matrix size is annotated by two figures. The first figure usually corresponds to the number of frequency samples taken, the second corresponds to the number of phase encodings performed. For example, 256 × 192 indicates that 256 frequency samples are taken during readout and 192 phase encodings are performed.

The more frequency samples taken and the more phase encodings that are performed, the more pixels there are in the FOV. A *coarse matrix* refers to a low number of pixels in the FOV, and a *fine matrix* refers to a high number of pixels in the FOV (Fig. 3.25).

To create an image, each pixel is allocated a signal intensity, corresponding to the amplitude of the signal originating from the anatomy at the position of each pixel in the matrix. Each pixel is allocated a signal intensity depending on the signal amplitude with a distinct frequency and phase shift pseudo-frequency value.

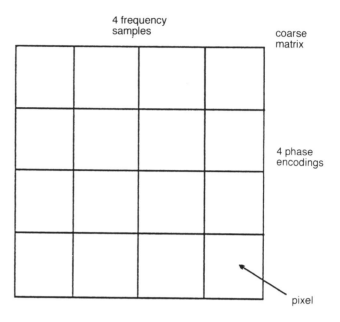

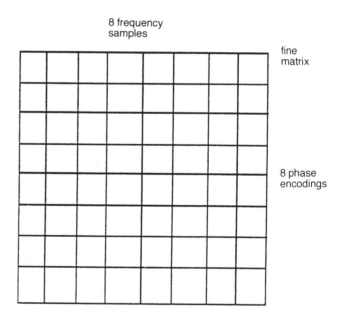

Fig. 3.25 The image matrix.

Data collection – Step 2

When all the lines of K space that have been selected are filled, the acquisition is over. The signal can be sampled more than once with the same slope of phase encoding gradient. Doing so, each line of K space is filled more than once. The number of times each signal is sampled with the same slope of phase encoding gradient is usually called *the number of signal averages (NSA)* or *the number of excitations (NEX)*. The higher the NEX, the more data that is stored in each line of K space. As there is more data stored in each line of K space, the amplitude of signal at each frequency and phase shift is greater (Fig. 3.26).

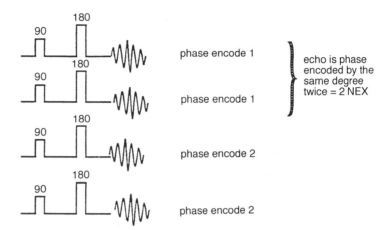

Fig. 3.26 Signal averaging.

Scan timing

Every TR each slice is selected, phase encoded and frequency encoded. The maximum number of slices that can be selected and encoded depends on the length of the TR, i.e. a longer TR allows more slices to be selected and encoded than a shorter TR. A TR of 500 ms may, for example, allow enough time for approximately 12 slices to be selected and encoded, whereas a TR of 2000 ms may only allow enough time for approximately 18 slices to be selected and encoded (Fig. 3.27).

The phase encoding gradient slope is altered every TR and is applied to each selected slice in order to phase encode it. At each phase encode a different line of K space is filled. The number of phase encoding steps therefore affects the length of the scan.

- If 128 phase encodings are selected, 128 lines are filled.
- If 256 phase encodings are selected, 256 lines are filled (Fig. 3.28).

As one phase encoding is performed each TR (to each slice):

- 128 phase encodings requires 128 × TR to complete the scan.
- 256 phase encodings requires 256 × TR to complete the scan.

If the TR is 1 s (1000 ms) the scan takes 128 s (if 128 phase encodings are performed) and 256 s (if 256 phase encodings are performed).

The scan time is also affected by the number of times the signal is phase encoded with the same phase encoding gradient slope, or NEX. If each

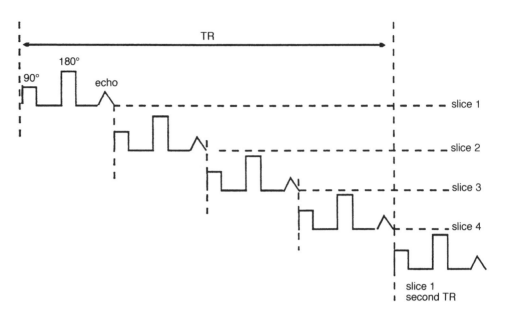

Fig. 3.27 TR versus number of slices. Note: the TR is the time between the 90° excitation pulse for each slice, not the time between successive excitation pulses.

signal is phase encoded with the same amplitude of phase encoding gradient slope twice, the TR must be repeated twice for each slope and therefore each line of K space. Therefore:

scan time = TR × number of phase encodings × NEX

K space filling

As previously discussed, K space can be represented diagramatically by a rectangle consisting of horizontal lines; the horizontal axis of K space is the phase axis, the vertical axis of K space is the frequency axis. At present, the maximum number of lines of K space on most systems is 1024. The lines of K space above the phase axis are termed positive, the lines of K space below the phase axis are termed negative. The negative half of K space is a mirror image of the positive half of K space, i.e. the data filling the positive half looks exactly the same as the negative half. The polarity of the phase gradient determines whether the positive or negative half of K space is filled. Gradient polarity depends on the direction of the current through the gradient coil.

The lines nearest to the phase axis both positively and negatively, are called the *central lines*. The central lines of K space are filled with data produced after the application of shallow phase encoding gradient slopes. The lines farthest away from the phase axis both positively and negatively, are called the *outer lines* of K space. These outer lines are filled with data produced after the application of the steep phase encoding gradient

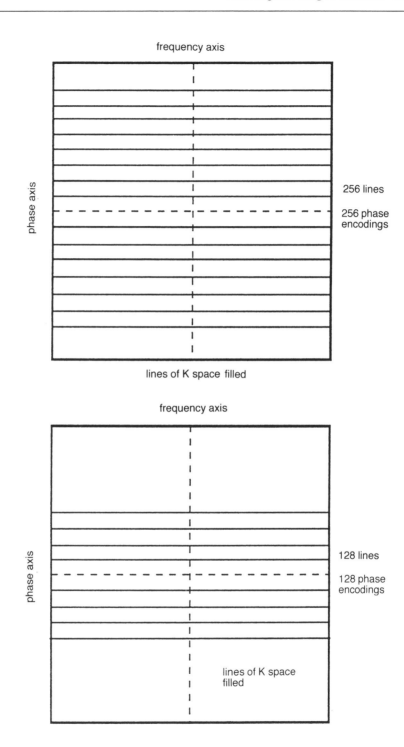

Fig. 3.28 The number of phase encoding steps and the lines of K space.

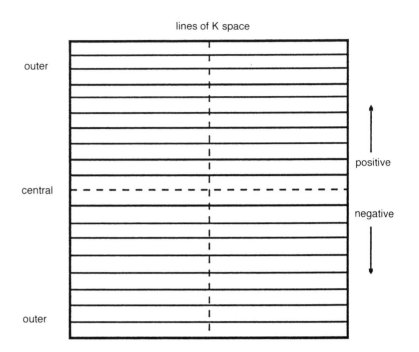

Fig. 3.29 The two halves of K space.

slopes. The lines in-between the central and outer portions, are filled with the intermediate phase encoding slopes (Fig. 3.29). The steepness of the slope of the phase gradient depends on how much current is driven through the gradient coil.

Positive gradient slopes fill lines in the positive half of K space, and negative gradients fill lines in the negative half. The central lines of K space are usually filled first so that if 256 phase encodings are performed for example, 128 positive and 128 negative lines of K space are filled on each side of the centre phase axis. If however 128 phase encodings are performed, the central 128 lines are filled (64 positive, 64 negative). The K space lines are usually filled sequentially, i.e. either from top to bottom, or from bottom to top (Fig. 3.30). However, K space can also be filled from the centre out (centric) or from the edges in.

K space filling and signal amplitude

As previously described, the central lines of K space are filled using the shallow phase encoding slopes, and the outer lines are filled using the steep phase encoding slopes. Shallow phase encoding slopes do not produce a large phase shift along their axis. The resultant signal therefore has a large amplitude. Steep phase encoding slopes produce a large phase shift along their axis. The resultant signal has a small amplitude (Fig. 3.31).

The vertical axis of K space corresponds to the frequency encoding axis. The area of K space to the left of the frequency axis is a mirror image of the area to the right of the frequency axis. The frequencies sampled in

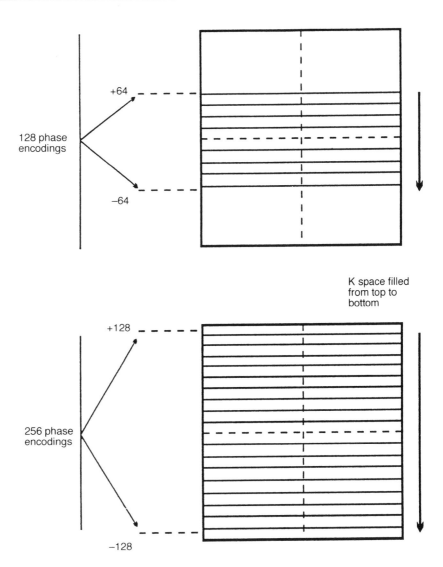

Fig. 3.30 K space filling.

the signal are mapped into K space relative to the frequency axis. The centre of the echo represents the maximum signal amplitude as all the magnetic moments are in phase, whereas the magnetic moments are either rephasing or dephasing on each side of the peak of the echo, and therefore the signal amplitude here is less. The amplitude of frequencies sampled is mapped relative to the frequency axis, so that the centre of the echo is placed central to the frequency axis. The rephasing and dephasing portions of the echo are mapped to the left and the right of the frequency axis (Fig. 3.32).

- The centre of K space contains data with the highest signal amplitude along both the phase and frequency axis.
- The outer portions of K space contain data with the lowest signal amplitude along both the phase and frequency axis.

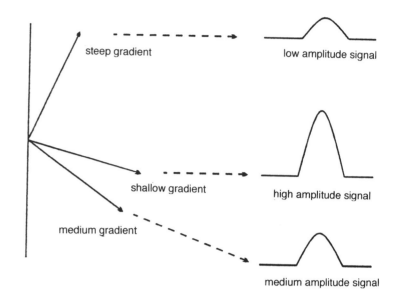

Fig. 3.31 The phase encoding slope versus signal amplitude.

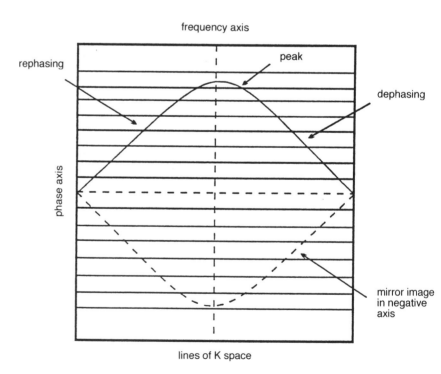

Fig. 3.32 The signal amplitude along the frequency axis.

K space filling and spatial resolution

The outer lines of K space contain data produced after steep phase encoding gradient slopes, and are only filled when many phase encodings have been performed. The number of phase encodings performed determines the number of pixels in the FOV along the phase encoding axis. When a large number of phase encodings are performed, there are more pixels in the FOV along the phase axis and therefore each pixel is smaller. If the FOV is fixed, voxels of smaller dimensions result in an image with a high spatial resolution, i.e. two points within the image can be distinguished more easily when the pixels are small (see Chapter 4). In addition, as the amplitude of the phase encoding gradient slope increases, the degree of phase shift along the gradient also increases. Two points adjacent to each other have a different phase value, and can therefore be differentiated from each other. Therefore, data collected after steep phase encoding gradient slopes produces greater spatial resolution in the image.

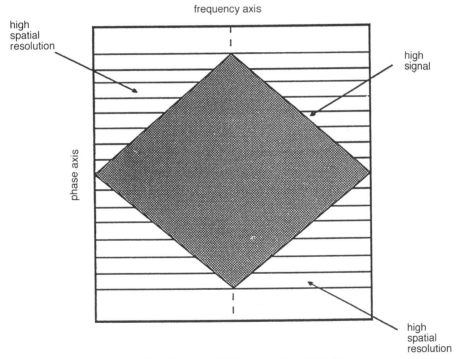

Fig. 3.33 K space – SNR and spatial resolution.

- The outer lines of K space contain data with a high spatial resolution as they are filled by steep phase encoding gradient slopes.
- The central lines of K space contain data with a low spatial resolution as they are filled by shallow phase encoding gradient slopes.

- The central portion of K space contains data that has high signal amplitude and low spatial resolution.
- The outer portion of K space contains data that has high spatial resolution and low signal amplitude (Fig. 3.33).

The way in which K space is traversed and filled depends on a combination of the polarity and amplitude of both the frequency and phase encoding gradients. The amplitude of the *frequency* encoding gradient determines how far to the *left and right* K space is traversed and this in turn determines the size of the FOV in the frequency direction of the image.

The amplitude of the *phase* encoding gradient determines how far *up and down* a line of K space is filled and in turn determines the size of the FOV in the phase direction of the image (or the spatial resolution when the FOV is square).

The polarity of each gradient defines the direction travelled through K space as follows:

- *frequency* encoding gradient *positive*, K space traversed *from left to right*,
- *frequency* encoding gradient *negative*, K space traversed *from right to left*,
- *phase* encoding gradient *positive*, fills *top* half of K space,
- *phase* encoding gradient *negative*, fills *bottom* half of K space.

This is best described using an illustration of a typical gradient echo sequence (Fig. 3.34). In a gradient echo sequence the frequency encoding gradient switches negatively to forcibly dephase the FID and then positively to rephase and produce a gradient echo (see Fig. 5.15). When the frequency encoding gradient is negative, K space is traversed from right to left. The starting point of K space filling is at the centre, so K space is initially traversed from the centre to the left, to a distance (A) which depends on the amplitude of the negative lobe of the frequency encoding gradient. The phase encode in this example is positive and therefore a line in the top half of K space is filled. The amplitude of this gradient determines the distance travelled (B). The larger the amplitude of the phase gradient, the higher up in K space is the line that is filled with data from the echo. Therefore the combination of the phase gradient and the negative lobe of the frequency gradient determines at what point in K space data storage begins.

The frequency encoding gradient is then switched positively and during its application data is read from the echo. As the frequency encoding gradient is positive, data is placed in a line of K space from left to right. The distance travelled depends on the amplitude of the positive lobe of the gradient and determines the size of the FOV (in this example we would expect the amplitude of the positive lobe to be twice that of the negative lobe because the distance travelled during readout is twice distance A).

This is only one example of how K space may be filled. If the phase

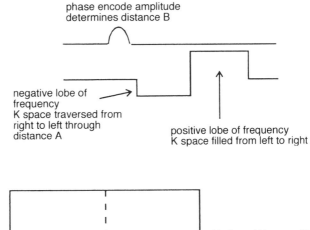

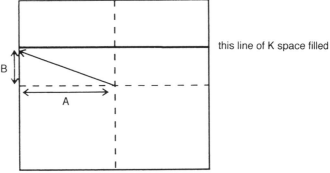

Fig. 3.34 K space traversal in gradient echo imaging.

gradient is negative then a line in the bottom half of K space is filled in exactly the same manner as above. K space traversal in spin echo sequences is more complex as the 180° RF pulse affects K space traversal dramatically. However, the principles are very similar.

The way in which K space is filled depends on how the data is acquired and can be manipulated to suit the circumstances of the scan. K space filling is manipulated in the following:

- rectangular field of view (Chapter 4),
- anti-aliasing (Chapter 7),
- ultra fast pulse sequences (Chapter 5),
- respiratory compensation (Chapter 7),
- echo planar imaging (Chapter 5).

The K space filling associated with the above options is discussed in the relevant chapters. However, it is appropriate here to describe two other options that use altered K space filling. These are:

(1) partial echo imaging,
(2) partial averaging.

Partial or fractional echo imaging

Partial echo imaging is performed when only part of the signal or echo is read during application of the frequency encoding gradient. As previously described, the peak of the echo or signal is usually centred in the middle of the readout gradient. For example, if the frequency encoding gradient is switched on for 8 ms, 4 ms of rephasing and 4 ms of dephasing is collected. This signal is mapped relative to the frequency axis of K space and one half the frequency area of K space is the mirror image of the other half. Therefore, data placed in one half of the frequency area of K space looks like that in the other half. If the system only samples half the echo, only half of the frequency area of K space is filled. However as the remaining is a mirror image, the system can calculate its amplitude accordingly. This filling of only half the area of K space along the frequency axis, is called *partial* or *fractional echo*. The echo no longer has to be centred on the middle of the frequency encoding gradient, as it can now occur at the beginning of the frequency encoding gradient application. In partial echo imaging the sampling window is shifted during readout so that only the peak and the dephasing part of the echo are sampled. As the peak of the echo can occur closer to the RF excitation pulse, the TE can be reduced when partial echo imaging is performed. In most systems, partial echo imaging is routinely used when a TE of less than 20 ms is selected. The use of a very short TE allows for maximum T1 and proton density weighting and slice number for a given TR (Fig. 3.35).

Partial or fractional averaging

The negative and positive halves of K space on each side of the phase axis are symmetrical and a mirror image of each other. As long as at least half of the lines of K space that have been selected are filled during the acquisition, the system has enough data to produce an image. If only 60% of K space is filled, only 60% of the phase encodings selected need to be performed to complete the scan, and the remaining lines are filled with zeros. The scan time is therefore reduced.
256 phase encodings, 1 NEX and TR of 1 s are selected.

$$\text{Scan time} = 256 \times 1 \times 1$$
$$= 256 \text{ s}$$

256 phase encodings, $\frac{3}{4}$ NEX and TR of 1 s are selected. Only 75% of K space is filled with data during the scan. The rest is filled with zeros (Fig. 3.36).

$$\text{Scan time} = 256 \times \tfrac{3}{4} \times 1$$
$$= 192 \text{ s}$$

The scan time is reduced but less data is acquired so the image has less signal. Partial averaging can be used where a reduction in scan time is necessary, and where the resultant signal loss is not of paramount importance.

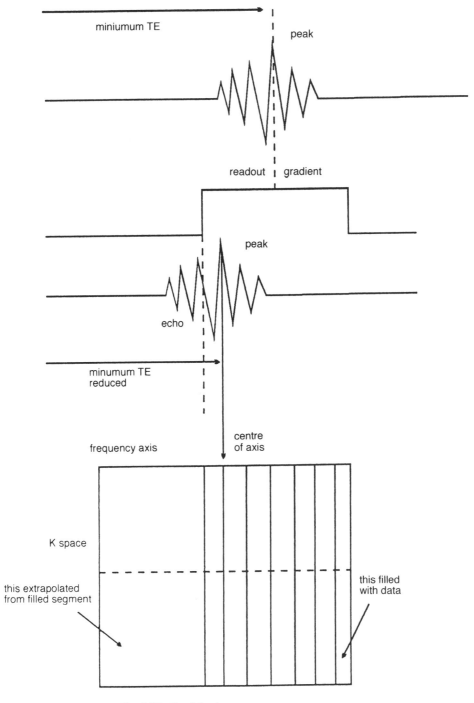

Fig. 3.35 Partial echo.

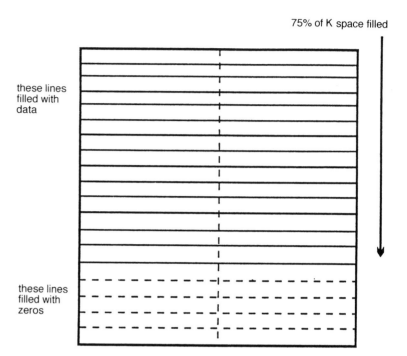

these lines filled with data

75% of K space filled

these lines filled with zeros

Fig. 3.36 Partial averaging.

PRE-SCAN

Pre-scanning is a method of calibration that should be performed before every data acquisition. Most systems perform automatic pre-scan procedures. However, there are occasions when this fails and so it is important that the various components of pre-scanning are understood. Every manufacturer performs pre-scan in a different manner. However, generally speaking the three main tasks that pre-scan performs are:

- Finding the centre frequency on which to transmit RF. This is usually chosen to be the resonant frequency of water protons within the area under examination, but can be adjusted to centre on the fat protons if required.
- Finding the exact magnitude of RF that must be transmitted to generate maximum signal in the coil. This is always equal to the energy required to flip the NMV through 90° into the transverse plane. From this, the system can calculate how much energy is required for flip angles other than 90°. This is known as the power spectrum or transmit gain.
- Adjustment of the magnitude of the received signal so that it is neither too large (which leads to distortion), nor that it is too small and cannot be properly detected above the background noise.

Pre-scan calculation varies with the type of pulse sequence used, the patient and the scan parameters chosen and it should be performed before every acquisition of data if image quality is to be optimised. Pre-scan may fail if:

(1) the coil is not plugged in properly,
(2) the coil is faulty,
(3) chemical saturation techniques are utilised and there is an uneven distribution of fat or water in the area to be saturated,
(4) the patient is either very large or very small.

Under these circumstances, the fault should be rectified if necessary and the pre-scan performed manually by the operator if possible.

Types of acquisition

There are basically three ways of acquiring data:

(1) sequential,
(2) two-dimensional volumetric,
(3) three-dimensional volumetric.

Sequential acquisitions acquire all the data from slice 1 and then go on to acquire all the data from slice 2, (all the lines in K space are filled for slice 1 and then all the lines of K space are filled for slice 2, etc.). The slices are therefore displayed as they are acquired (not unlike computerised tomography scanning).

Two-dimensional volumetric acquisitions fill one line of K space for slice 1, and then go on to fill the same line of K space for slice 2, etc. When this line has been filled for all the slices, the next line of K space is filled for slice 1, 2, 3, etc.

LEARNING POINT

An easy analogy is to imagine three glasses which must be filled with water. Each glass represents a slice, and the water represents data. Sequential acquisition corresponds to filling all of glass 1 with water before filling glass 2. Two-dimensional volumetric acquisition corresponds to pouring a small amount of water into glass 1 and then into glasses 2 and 3. The pourer then returns to glass 1 and pours a small amount in again, and so on. When all the glasses are full, or when all the lines of K space have been filled for each slice, the acquisition is over and the slices are displayed (Fig. 3.37).

Three-dimensional volumetric acquisition (volume imaging) acquires data from an entire volume of tissue, rather than in separate slices. The excitation pulse is not slice selective, and the whole prescribed imaging volume is excited. At the end of the acquisition the volume or slab is divided into discrete locations or partitions by the slice select gradient that, when switched on, separates the slices according to their phase value along the gradient. This process is now called slice encoding. Many slices

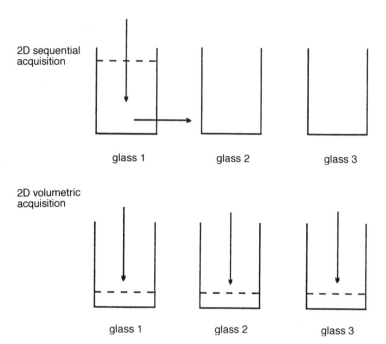

Fig. 3.37 Data acquisition – the glass analogy.

can be obtained, (typically 28, 64, or 128) without a slice gap. In other words the slices are contiguous. The advantages of volume imaging are discussed in more detail in Chapter 4.

This chapter has introduced the basic mechanisms of gradients. A more detailed discussion, including high speed gradient systems and their applications, is to be found in Chapter 12.

As data acquisition and image formation have now been explored, the parameters available to the operator and how they interact with each other are described in the next chapter.

Questions

1. Name three gradient functions.

2. What controls the polarity of a gradient?

3. What factor does the frequency encoding gradient slope control?

4. What operator function alters the number of pixels in the image?

5. What is K space?

6. Define the Nyquist theorem.

7. How is K space filling altered in the following:
   (a) partial echo?
   (b) fractional echo?

Chapter 4   Parameters and Trade-offs

Introduction

There are many parameters available to the operator when setting up a sequence. The choice of pulse sequence determines the weighting and the quality of the images as well as their sensitivity to pathology. The timing parameters selected specifically determine the weighting of the images.

- TR determines the amount of T1 and proton density weighting.
- Flip angle controls the amount of T1 and proton density weighting.
- TE controls the amount of T2 weighting.

The quality of the images is controlled by many factors. It is very important that the operator is aware of these factors and how they interrelate, so that the optimal image quality can always be obtained. The four main considerations determining image quality are:

(1) signal to noise ratio (SNR),
(2) contrast to noise ratio (CNR),
(3) spatial resolution,
(4) scan time.

Signal to noise ratio (SNR)

This is the ratio of the amplitude of the signal received to the average amplitude of the noise. The signal is the voltage induced in the receiver coil by the precession of the NMV in the transverse plane. The noise is generated by the presence of the patient in the magnet, and the background electrical noise of the system. The noise is constant for every patient and depends on the build of the patient, the area under examination and the inherent noise of the system. Noise occurs at all frequencies and is also random in time. The signal however, is cumulative and depends on many factors and can be altered. The signal is therefore increased or decreased relative to the noise. Increasing the signal increases the SNR, whilst decreasing the signal decreases the SNR. Therefore, any factor that affects the signal amplitude in turn affects the SNR. The factors that affect the SNR are:

- proton density of the area under examination,
- voxel volume,
- TR, TE and flip angle,
- NEX,
- receive bandwidth,
- coil type.

Proton density

The number of protons in the area under examination determines the amplitude of signal received. Areas of low proton density (such as the lungs), have low signal and therefore low SNR, whereas areas with a high proton density (such as the pelvis), have high signal and therefore high SNR.

Voxel volume

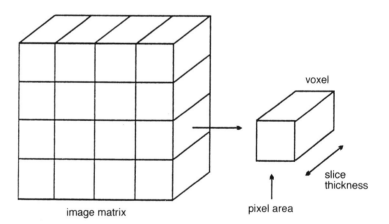

Fig. 4.1 The voxel.

The building unit of a digital image is a pixel. The brightness of the pixel represents the strength of the MRI signal generated by a unit volume of patient tissue or voxel. The *voxel* represents a volume of tissue within the patient, and is determined by the pixel area and the slice thickness (Fig. 4.1). The pixel area is determined by the size of the FOV and the number of pixels in the FOV or matrix. Therefore:

$$\text{pixel area} = \frac{\text{FOV dimensions}}{\text{matrix size}}$$

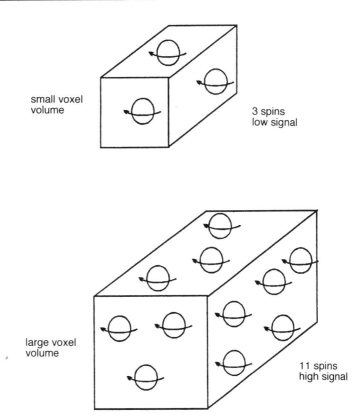

small voxel
volume

3 spins
low signal

large voxel
volume

11 spins
high signal

Fig. 4.2 Voxel volume and
SNR. (Spin numbers are not
representative.)

A coarse matrix is one with a low number of frequency encodings and/or
phase encodings and results in a low number of pixels in the FOV. A
coarse matrix results in large pixels and voxels (assuming a given square
FOV). A fine matrix is one where there are a high number of frequency
encodings and/or phase encodings, and results in a large number of pixels
in the FOV. A fine matrix results in small pixels and voxels. Large voxels
contain more spins or nuclei than small voxels, and therefore have more
nuclei within them to contribute towards the signal. Large voxels have a
higher SNR than small voxels (Fig. 4.2).

The SNR is therefore proportional to the voxel volume and any
parameter that alters the size of the voxel changes the SNR. Any selection
that decreases the size of the voxel decreases the SNR, and vice versa.
The voxel is altered by a change in the slice thickness or the pixel area.
Doubling the slice thickness doubles the voxel volume and the SNR, whilst
halving the slice thickness halves the SNR (Fig. 4.3).

The pixel area is altered by changing the matrix size or the FOV.
Assuming that the FOV remains square, doubling the number of phase
encodings, halves the pixel dimension along the phase axis. This halves
the voxel volume and the SNR. The opposite is true when halving the
number of phase encodings – the voxel volume, and the SNR double.

Doubling the FOV doubles the voxel volume along both axes of the

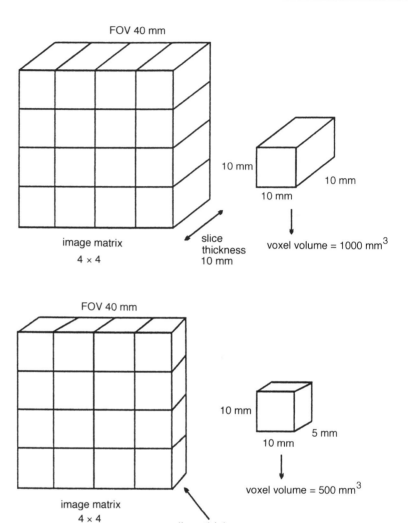

Fig. 4.3 Slice thickness versus SNR.

pixel, and increases the voxel volume and SNR fourfold. The opposite is true when halving the FOV – the voxel volume and the SNR are reduced to a quarter of their original value. The FOV is therefore one of the most potent factors affecting the SNR (Fig. 4.4).

TR, TE and flip angle

Although TR, TE and flip angle are usually considered as parameters that influence image contrast, they also influence the SNR and therefore overall image quality. Spin echo pulse sequences generally have more signal than gradient echo sequences, as all the longitudinal magnetisation is converted into transverse magnetisation by the 90° flip angle. Gradient echo pulse sequences only convert a proportion of the longitudinal

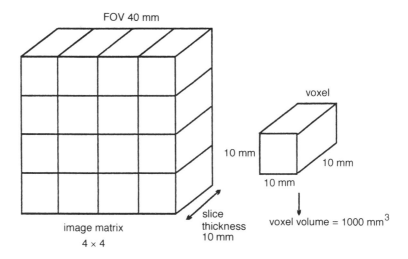

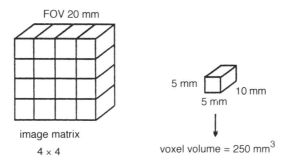

Fig. 4.4 FOV versus SNR.

magnetisation into transverse magnetisation, as they use flip angles other than 90°. In addition, the 180° rephasing pulse is more efficient at rephasing than the rephasing gradient of gradient echo sequences, and so the resultant echo has a greater signal amplitude.

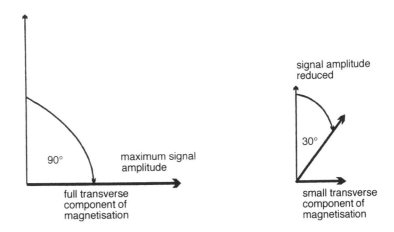

Fig. 4.5 Flip angle versus SNR.

The flip angle controls the amount of transverse magnetisation that is created which induces a signal in the coil (Fig. 4.5). The maximum signal amplitude is created with flip angles of 90°.

The lower the flip angle, the lower the SNR.

The TR controls the amount of longitudinal magnetisation that is allowed to recover before the next excitation pulse is applied. A long TR allows full recovery of the longitudinal magnetisation so that more is available to be flipped in the next repetition. A short TR does not allow full recovery of longitudinal magnetisation, so less is available to be flipped.

A long TR increases SNR and a short TR reduces SNR.

The TE controls the amount of transverse magnetisation that is allowed to decay before an echo is collected. A long TE allows considerable decay of the transverse magnetisation to occur before the echo is collected, whilst a short TE does not (Fig. 4.6).

A long TE reduces SNR and a short TE increases SNR.

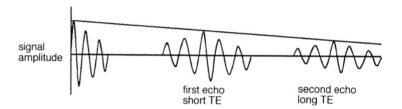

Fig. 4.6 TE versus SNR.

Number of averages (NEX)

This is the number of times data is collected with the same amplitude of phase encoding slope. The NEX controls the amount of data that is stored in each line of K space. Doubling the NEX therefore doubles the amount of data that is stored in each line of K space, whereas halving the NEX halves the amount of data stored. The data contains both signal and noise. Noise is random as it is in a different position each time data is stored. Signal however is not random, as it always occurs at the same place when it is collected. The presence of random noise means that doubling the NEX only increases the SNR by $\sqrt{2}$ (= 1.4). Therefore increasing the NEX, is not necessarily the best way of increasing SNR (Fig. 4.7).

Increasing the NEX also reduces motion artefact. This is discussed later in the book.

Receive bandwidth

This is the range of frequencies that are sampled during the application of the readout gradient. Reducing the receive bandwidth results in less noise

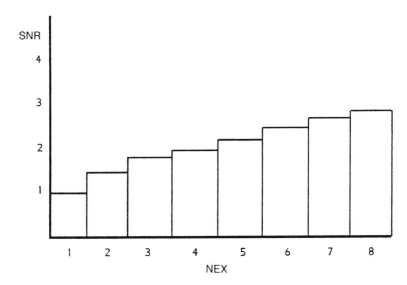

Fig. 4.7   NEX versus SNR.

being sampled relative to signal. As less noise is sampled as a proportion of signal, the SNR increases as the receive bandwidth decreases (Fig. 4.8). Halving the bandwidth increases the SNR by about 40%, but increases the sampling time as the Nyquist theorem must be obeyed. As a result, reducing the bandwidth increases the minimum TE available (see Chapter 3). Reducing the bandwidth also increases chemical shift artefact (see Chapter 7).

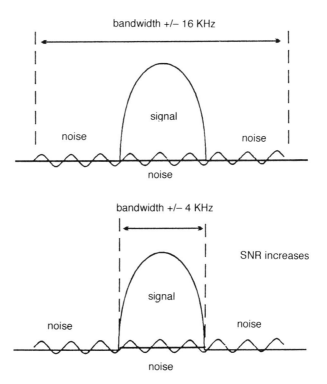

Fig. 4.8   Bandwidth versus SNR.

Type of coil

The type of coil used affects the amount of signal received and therefore the SNR. Coil types are discussed in Chapter 9. Quadrature coils increase SNR as two coils are used to receive signal. Surface coils placed close to the area under examination also increase the SNR. The use of the appropriate receiver coil plays an extremely important role in optimising SNR.

In general, the size of the receiver coil should be chosen such that the volume of tissue imaged optimally fills the sensitive volume of the coil. Large coils, however, increase the likelihood of aliasing as tissue outside the FOV is more likely to produce signal.

How to increase SNR

To optimise image quality the SNR must be the highest possible. To achieve this:

- use spin echo pulse sequences where possible,
- try not to use a very short TR and a very long TE,
- use the correct coil and ensure that it is well tuned,
- use a coarse matrix,
- use a large FOV,
- select thick slices,
- use as many NEX as possible.

Contrast to noise ratio (CNR)

This is defined as the difference in the SNR between two adjacent areas. It is controlled by the same factors that affect SNR. The CNR is probably the most critical factor affecting image quality as it directly determines the eyes' ability to distinguish areas of high signal from areas of low signal. For example, although a T2 weighted image often has a much lower SNR than a T1 weighted image (due to the longer TE), the ability to distinguish tumour from normal tissue is often much greater because of the high signal of the tumour compared to the low signal of surrounding anatomy, i.e. the CNR is higher. Indeed the purpose of administering contrast agents is to increase the CNR between pathology (which enhances) and normal anatomy (which does not) (see Chapter 11).

Image contrast depends on the following:

- TR
- TE
- TI
- flip angle
- flow

- turbo factor (in fast spin echo)
- T1
- T2
- proton density.

Another technique that affects the CNR between tissues is magnetisation transfer.

In MRI, only protons that have a sufficiently long T2 time can be imaged. Other protons whose transverse components decay before the signal can be collected cannot be visualised adequately. These protons, mainly bound to large proteins, membranes, and other macro-molecules are called bound protons. The protons that have longer T2 times can be visualised and are termed free protons. There is always a transfer of magnetisation between the bound and the free protons which causes a change in the T1 values of the free protons. This can be exploited by selectively saturating the bound protons which reduces the intensity of the signal from the free protons due to magnetisation transfer coherence (MTC). The MTC saturation band is applied before the excitation pulse at a bandwidth that selectively destroys the transverse components of magnetisation of the bound protons. The use of MTC increases the CNR between pathological and normal tissues and is useful in many areas including angiography and joint imaging.

Spatial resolution

The spatial resolution is the ability to distinguish between two points as separate and distinct, and is controlled by the voxel size. Small voxels result in good spatial resolution as small structures can be easily differentiated. Large voxels, on the other hand, result in low spatial resolution, as small structures are not resolved so well. In large voxels, individual signal intensities are averaged together and not represented as distinct within the voxel. This results in partial voluming. The voxel size is affected by:

(1) slice thickness,
(2) FOV,
(3) number of pixels or matrix.

The thinner the slice, the greater the ability to resolve small structures in the slice select plane. Reducing the slice thickness therefore increases spatial resolution, whereas increasing the slice thickness reduces spatial resolution and increases *partial voluming*.

The matrix determines the number of pixels in the FOV. Small pixels increase spatial resolution as they increase the ability to distinguish between two structures close together in the patient. Increasing the matrix therefore increases the spatial resolution (Fig. 4.9).

The size of the FOV also determines the pixel dimensions. A large FOV

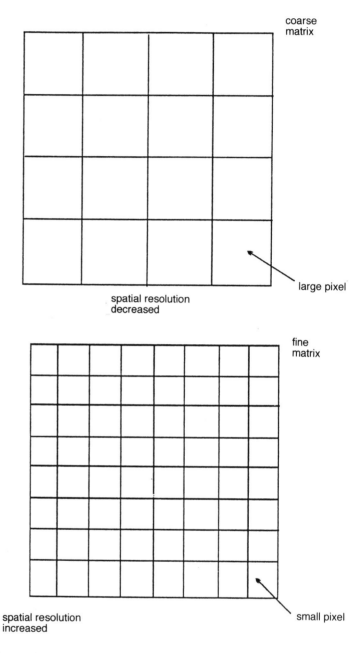

Fig. 4.9 Pixel size versus matrix size.

results in large pixels, whereas a small FOV produces small pixels. Increasing the FOV size therefore decreases the spatial resolution.

Spatial resolution and pixel dimension

Square pixels always provide better spatial resolution than rectangular pixels as the image is equally resolved along both the frequency and phase axis. If the FOV is square, the pixels are also square if an even matrix is selected, e.g. 256 × 256. If the FOV is square and an uneven matrix is selected, for example, 256 × 128, the pixels are rectangular.

Usually, the frequency number of the matrix is the highest number and the phase number is altered to change the scan time and the resolution. If the phase number is less than the frequency number, the pixels are longer in the phase direction than in the frequency direction. The spatial resolution is therefore reduced along the phase axis. Some systems however, automatically keep the pixels square regardless of the matrix selected. Therefore, if the number of phase encodings is half that of the frequency encodings, the FOV in the phase direction is half the size that it is in the frequency direction, but the pixels remain square. This method maintains the spatial resolution regardless of the matrix selected (Fig. 4.10).

However, the FOV should always cover the required anatomy along the phase axis. To increase the FOV in the phase direction, the number of

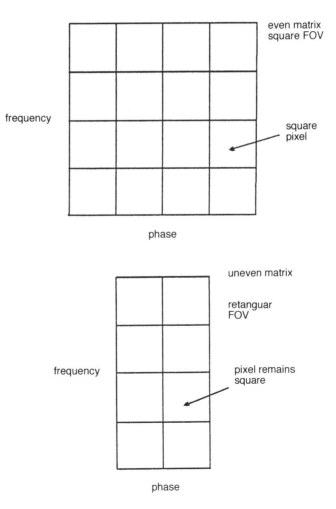

Fig. 4.10 Square pixels.

phase encodings must be increased, and this increases the scan time. In addition, the SNR from the smaller square pixels is lower than with rectangular pixels. Systems that employ this method usually have the option of selecting rectangular pixels, which automatically keeps the FOV square, so that the anatomy in the phase direction is covered and the SNR increased. This is achieved without increasing the phase encoding number (and therefore the scan time), as the pixels are automatically made rectangular in the phase direction. Although the spatial resolution is reduced, the SNR increases as each pixel is now larger (Fig. 4.11).

- Square pixels   maintain SNR regardless of the matrix chosen. The matrix determines the scan time and the FOV.
- Rectangular pixels   maintain a square FOV regardless of the matrix chosen. The matrix determines the scan time and the resolution.

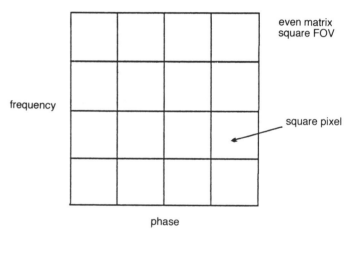

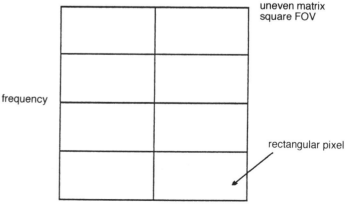

Fig. 4.11 Rectangular pixels.

Many systems always use this latter method of keeping the FOV square. In these systems, the matrix size governs the spatial resolution and SNR, as well as scan time. These systems have an option called *rectangular FOV* to maintain spatial resolution with an uneven matrix.

Rectangular FOV

In some cases, where the system allows for rectangular pixels but the anatomy does not fill a square FOV, a rectangular FOV may be desired. To acquire a square FOV, high resolution image is costly in time. For this purpose many systems offer an option known as rectangular FOV.

Rectangular FOV maintains spatial resolution but halves the scan time as only half the number of phase encodings that are normally required are performed. The dimension of the FOV in the phase direction is half that of the frequency direction and so should be used when imaging anatomy that fits into a rectangle, for example, a sagittal lumbar spine image. If rectangular FOV is selected with a 256×256 matrix and 24 cm FOV, the resolution of 256×256 is maintained but the scan is completed after only 128 phase encodings. The FOV is 24 cm in the frequency direction and 12 cm in the phase direction.

Rectangular FOV and K space filling

If a 256×256 matrix has been selected, 128 positive and 128 negative K space lines must normally be filled: 256 phase encodings therefore have to be performed to finish the scan. In rectangular FOV, the resolution of 256 phase encodings must be achieved, and so the very steepest phase encoding gradient slopes at $+128$ and -128 should still be performed. However, the scan should just take the time to apply 128 phase encodings. To achieve this, only 128 phase encodings between $+128$ and -128 are performed. The increment between each phase encoding step is therefore doubled. The phase increments are the difference in angle between successive phase encoding slopes. The size of the phase increment is inversely proportional to the size of the FOV in the phase direction. Therefore if the phase increment is halved, the FOV in the phase direction doubles and vice versa. In rectangular FOV, the phase increment is doubled so that only 128 phase encodings need to be performed between $+128$ and -128, and therefore the size of the FOV is halved in the phase direction (Fig. 4.12).

How to increase spatial resolution

To improve image quality the spatial resolution must be optimised. The spatial resolution can be maintained by:

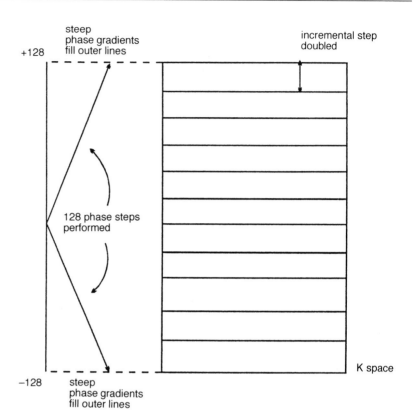

Fig. 4.12 Rectangular FOV and K space filling.

- selecting as thin a slice as possible,
- selecting a fine matrix,
- selecting a small FOV,
- selecting rectangular FOV where possible.

LEARNING POINT

The slice thickness is determined by the slope of the slice select gradient. Therefore, to achieve *thin slices* the slice select gradient slope is STEEP. The size of the FOV is determined by the slope of the frequency encoding gradient. To achieve a *small FOV*, the frequency encoding gradient slope is STEEP. The matrix size in the phase direction is determined by the number of phase encodings performed. To achieve a *fine matrix* a high proportion of the phase encoding gradient slopes are STEEP.

If gradient slopes have to be steep during a pulse sequence because thin slices, fine matrices or a small FOV has been selected, their rise times are greater. The *rise time* of a gradient is the time required for it to achieve the correct slope. Steep gradient slopes result in a higher rise time for the gradient than shallow gradient slopes. Steep gradient slopes therefore stress the gradient coils more than shallow gradient slopes. This therefore, increases the minimum TE as the system is not ready to collect the signal until all the gradient functions have been achieved. A small FOV, thin slices and fine matrices increase the minimum TE and may result in fewer slices being available. If the TE increases, the selection and encoding of each slice takes longer, and therefore less slices can be excited in a given TR.

Scan time

The scan time is the time to complete data acquisition. Scan times are important in maintaining image quality, as long scan times give the patient more of a chance to move during the acquisition. Any movement of the patient will probably degrade the images. As multiple slices are selected during a 2D and 3D volumetric acquisition, movement during these types of acquisition affects all the slices. During a sequential acquisition, movement of the patient only affects those slices that are acquired while the patient is moving.

The factors that affect scan time are:

(1) TR,
(2) number of phase encodings,
(3) NEX.

The TR is the time of each repetition or MR experiment. Doubling the TR doubles the scan time and vice versa. The number of phase encodings determines the number of lines of K space that are filled to complete the scan. If the number of phase encodings are doubled, the scan time also doubles. The NEX is the number of times data is collected with the same slope of phase encoding gradient. Doubling the NEX doubles the scan time and vice versa.

How to reduce the scan time

To reduce the likelihood of patient movement, the scan time should always be as short as possible. To achieve the shortest scan time:

(1) use the shortest TR possible,
(2) select the coarsest matrix possible,
(3) reduce the NEX to a minimum.

Figures 4.13 to 4.16 show sagittal images of the brain obtained using different parameters.

- SNR is proportional to:
  pixel area/FOV^2,
  slice thickness,
  proton density,
  $\sqrt{NEX}$,
  $1/\sqrt{}$(number of phase encodings),
  $1/\sqrt{}$(number of frequency encodings),
  $1/\sqrt{}$ (receive bandwidth),
  TR, TE and flip angle.

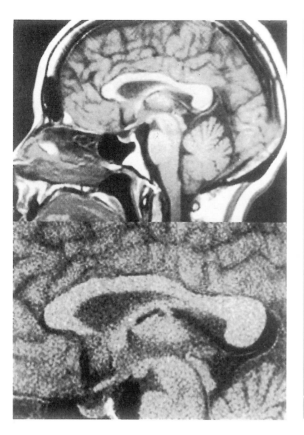

Fig. 4.13 Sagittal T1 weighted images of the brain using an FOV of 24 cm (above) and 12 cm (below). The lower image has greater spatial resolution, but a much reduced SNR.

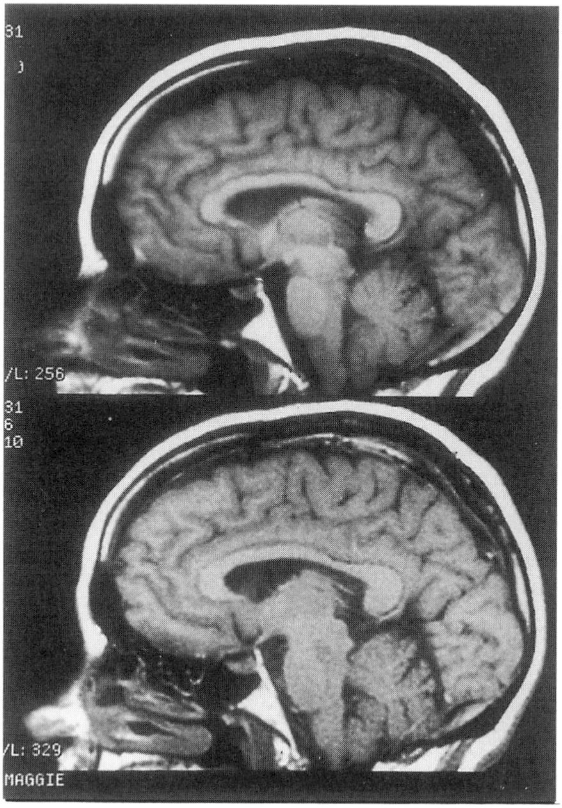

Fig. 4.14 Sagittal T1 weighted images of the brain with a 10 mm slice thickness (above) and a 3 mm slice thickness (below). The lower image has greater resolution but a lower SNR.

- Spatial resolution is determined by:
    FOV,
    matrix size,
    slice thickness.
- Scan time is proportional to:
    TR,
    number of phase encodings,
    NEX.

Trade-offs

It is probably now obvious that there are many trade-offs when selecting parameters within a pulse sequence. Ideally an image has high SNR, good spatial resolution and is acquired in a very short scan time. However, this is rarely achievable as increasing one factor, inevitably reduces one or both of the other two. It is vital that the user has a full understanding of all

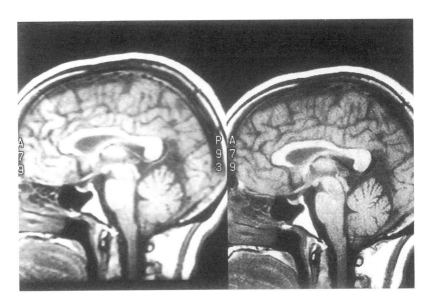

Fig. 4.15 Sagittal images of the brain. The image on the left was acquired with a matrix of 256 × 128, whereas the image on the right was acquired with a matrix of 512 × 256. The image on the right demonstrates improved spatial resolution. Which image took longer to acquire?

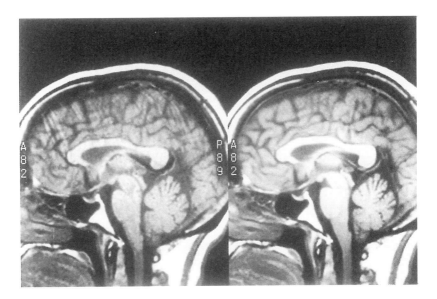

Fig. 4.16 Sagittal images of the brain. The image on the left used partial averaging and took 56 s to acquire. The image on the right, used 4 signal averages and took 6 min to acquire, (all other parameters remained constant). The image on the right has a greater SNR than the left.

the parameters that affect each image quality parameter and the trade-offs involved. Table 4.1 gives the result of optimising image quality. Table 4.2 gives the parameters and their associated trade-offs.

Table 4.1 The results of optimising image quality.

To optimise image	Adjusted parameter	Consequence
Maximise SNR	↑ NEX	↑ scan time
	↓ matrix	↓ scan time ↓ spatial resolution
	↑ slice thickness	↓ spatial resolution
	↓ receive bandwidth	↑ minimum TE ↑ chemical shift
	↑ FOV	↓ spatial resolution
	↑ TR	↓ T1 weighting ↑ number of slices
	↓ TE	↓ T2 weighting
Maximise spatial resolution	↓ slice thickness	↓ SNR
(assuming a square FOV)	↑ matrix	↓ SNR ↑ scan time
	↓ FOV	↓ SNR
Minimise scan time	↓ TR	↑ T1 weighting ↓ SNR ↓ number of slices
	↓ phase encodings	↓ spatial resolution ↑ SNR
	↓ NEX	↑ SNR ↑ movement artefact
	↓ slice number in volume imaging	↓ SNR

Decision making

The decisions made when setting up a pulse sequence depend on the area to be examined, the condition and co-operation of the patient and the clinical throughput required. There are really no rules in MRI – this can be very frustrating when trying to learn, but also makes the subject interesting and challenging. Every facility has protocols established with the co-operation of the manufacturer and the radiologist. However, here are a few tips for optimising image quality.

Table 4.2 Parameters and their associated trade-offs.

Parameter	Benefit	Limitation
TR increased	increased SNR increased number of slices	increased scan time decreased T1 weighting
TR decreased	decreased scan time increased T1 weighting	decreased SNR decreased number of slices
TE increased	increased T2 weighting	decreased SNR
TE decreased	increased SNR	decreased T2 weighting
NEX increased	increased SNR more signal averaging	direct proportional increase in scan time
NEX decreased	direct proportional decrease in scan time	decreased SNR less signal averaging
Slice thickness increased	increased SNR increased coverage of anatomy	decreased spatial resolution more partial voluming
Slice thickness decreased	increased spatial resolution reduced partial voluming	decreased SNR decreased coverage of anatomy
FOV increased	increased SNR increased coverage of anatomy	decreased spatial resolution decreased likelihood of aliasing
FOV decreased	increased spatial resolution increased likelihood of aliasing	decreased SNR decreased coverage of anatomy
Matrix increased	increased spatial resolution	increased scan time decreased SNR if pixel is small
Matrix decreased	decreased scan time increased SNR if pixel is large	decreased spatial resolution
Receive bandwidth increased	decrease in chemical shift decrease in minimum TE	decreased SNR
Receive bandwidth decreased	increased SNR	increase in chemical shift increase in minimum TE
Large coil	increased area of received signal	lower SNR sensitive to artefacts aliasing with small FOV
Small coil	increased SNR less sensitive to artefacts less prone to aliasing with a small FOV	decreased area of received signal

- Always choose the correct coil. This often makes the difference between a good or bad quality examination.
- Make sure that the patient is comfortable. This is very important as a patient is more likely to move if he or she is uncomfortable. Immobilise the patient as much as possible to reduce the likelihood of movement.
- Try to ascertain from the radiologist exactly what sequences are required before the scan. This saves a lot of time as radiologists can be difficult to track down!
- The scan plane, pulse sequence type, and weighting required are usually (but not always) decided by the radiologist. In our view, SNR is the most important image quality factor. There is no point in having an image with good spatial resolution if the SNR is poor. Sometimes however, good spatial resolution is vital but if the SNR is low, the images will be of poor quality and the benefit of good spatial resolution is lost.
- It is very important to keep the scan time as short as possible. Again, there is no point having an image with great SNR and spatial resolution, if it took so long to acquire that the patient has moved during the scan. Remember, any patient can move – not just a restless one. The longer the patient is expected to lie on the table, the more likely it is that he or she will move.
- As each system varies considerably, the following are only guidelines. The parameters given are not etched in stone but are only meant as indicators. It is inadvisable to select:

> a very short TR (choose 400 not 200 ms),
> a very long TE (choose 100 not 200 ms),
> very low flip angles (choose 20° not 5°),
> very thin slices (choose 4 not 3 mm),
> a very small FOV (choose 12 not 8 cm), unless
> you are using a good local coil.

In most centres, the protocols selected work well and the radiologists are happy with the parameters set. However, it is worth remembering that a 1 mm difference for example in slice thickness, can make all the difference in improving SNR, without noticeably reducing the spatial resolution. Also remember that as the FOV size decreases, the dimensions of the pixel along both axes are reduced (assuming that the system operates with a square FOV). Under these circumstances, the FOV is the most potent controller of SNR. Using a 16 cm FOV instead of an 8 cm FOV, can be important in maintaining SNR. If the area under examination has inherently good signal (for example, the brain) and the correct coil has been selected, it is usually possible for a fine matrix and fewer NEX to be used to achieve good quality images in terms of SNR and spatial resolution. However when examining an area with inherently low signal (for example, the lungs), selection of more NEX and a coarser matrix may be necessary. Try to do all this and keep the scan time as low as possible. It is usually not practical to have sequences that last 30 min each!

Volume imaging

Volume imaging is advantageous in that very small lesions can be demonstrated, as the slice thickness can be drastically reduced compared with conventional imaging, and there is no slice gap. In conventional imaging the slice thickness affects the SNR. In volume imaging the entire volume of tissue is excited and the volume contains no gap, the SNR is superior, and so fewer NEX can be used. The other main advantage of volumes is that, as data is collected from a slab, the slab can be manipulated to look at the anatomy within the volume in any plane and at any angle of obliquity. The disadvantages of volume imaging are that, in general, the scan times associated with them are relatively long. For this reason, they are usually used in conjunction with faster pulse sequences. In volume imaging slices are sectioned out by a technique known as slice encoding. This is another series of phase encoding steps along the slice select axis. Therefore, just as the number of phase encoding steps increases the scan time in conventional spin echo, the number of slices also affects the scan time in volume imaging. Therefore:

$$\text{scan time} = \text{TR} \times \text{NEX} \times \text{number of phase encodings} \times \\ \text{number of slice encodings}$$

The greater the number of slices prescribed, the longer the scan time. However, this is off-set somewhat by the fact that the greater the slice number the greater the SNR, and so the NEX can be reduced (Fig. 4.17).

Volume imaging and resolution

To obtain equal resolution in *every* plane and at *every* angle of obliquity, each voxel should be symmetrical (*isotropic*). That is to say, that the voxel should have equal dimensions in every plane. If this is not true, the volume has poorer resolution in the planes other than the one in which it was acquired. For example, if a FOV of 24 cm and matrix of 256 × 256 is used, each pixel has a dimension of 0.9 mm (FOV/matrix). If the slice thickness selected is 3 mm, resolution is worse when the voxel is viewed from the side. Under these conditions, the voxel is *anisotropic*.

Sometimes volumes are acquired purely because the slices are contiguous and not because they are to be viewed in another plane, for example, coronal volumes of the brain can be very useful in detecting small temporal lobe lesions. However, they are not generally used to look at the brain axially or coronally. In this instance, 3 mm slices at 64 locations will cover the head adequately. In volume imaging of a joint on the other hand, reformatting in other planes may be paramount. Under these circumstances it is important to obtain isotropic voxels, so thinner slices (1 mm or less) are required, although the number of slice locations may have to be increased to cover the anatomy.

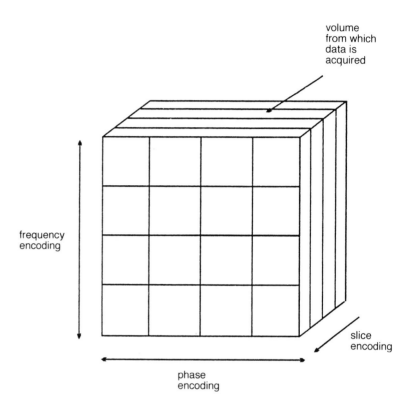

volume
from which
data is
acquired

frequency
encoding

slice
encoding

phase
encoding

Fig. 4.17 Encoding in a
volume acquisition.

The uses of volume imaging

Volume imaging has many potential applications, but it is widely used for
imaging of joints especially the knee, where anatomy is often confusing
and not strictly in plane. Volumes can be very useful for following
ligaments or other structures that cross over the imaging plane. Volumes
should also be used when looking for very small lesions. The slice
thickness can be lowered to less than 1 mm in most systems, and so
extremely good resolution can be achieved. Lesions in the temporal lobes
or posterior fossa especially lend themselves to volume imaging.

- Volume imaging allows reformatting in any plane.
- Isotropic voxels give equal resolution in every plane.
- The scan time depends on the slice number as well as the TR, phase
  encoding number and the NEX.
- Increasing the slice number increases the SNR, but also increases the
  scan time.
- Volume imaging increases the SNR as a whole volume of tissue is
  excited.

Manipulating SNR, image contrast, spatial resolution and scan time is a
real art and takes some time and experience. Even after many years the
operator will probably get things wrong occasionally! However, persever-

ance is important, and eventually results in good image quality. As image quality factors and trade-offs have been explored, it is now important to understand pulse sequences and their individual uses. This is discussed in Chapter 5.

Questions

1. Define spatial resolution.

2. Of the following parameters which would give:
   (a) the best spatial resolution?
   (b) the highest SNR?
   >   256 × 256, 3 mm slice thickness, 12 cm FOV, 1 NEX,
   >   256 × 128, 8 mm slice thickness, 40 cm FOV, 4 NEX,
   >   512 × 256, 4 mm slice thickness, 8 cm FOV, 2 NEX.

3. List three ways of improving the CNR between pathology and normal tissue.

4. You are examining a 90-year-old claustrophobic patient's cervical spine using the following parameters. The images you obtain are very noisy and have poor SNR. What factors would you change, and why?
   Body coil
   TR 700 ms a long TE
   16 slices
   256 × 128
   1 NEX
   FOV 12 cm
   3 mm slice thickness 1 mm gap.

5. How is K space filling altered in rectangular FOV?

6. What advantages does volume imaging have over normal slice acquisition?

7. How would you achieve equal resolution in all reformatting planes in a volume acquisition?

Chapter 5   Pulse Sequences

Introduction

Understanding pulse sequences forms an integral part of learning MRI. Pulse sequences enable us to control the way in which the system applies pulses and gradients. In this way, image weighting and quality is determined. There are many different pulse sequences available, and each is designed for a specific purpose. This chapter discusses the physics, uses and parameters for each of the common pulse sequences, as well as their advantages and disadvantages. Each manufacturer uses different acronyms to distinguish between individual pulse sequences, which can be very confusing to the user. A table comparing the common acronyms for each of the main manufacturers is included. This is provided as a guide only; it is not in any way meant to compare the performance, or specification of each system. An omission from the table indicates only that information about a certain factor was unavailable, not necessarily that it is not an option. The parameters given are very general, and each system will use variations of these. Pulse sequences can generally be categorised as follows:

- Spin echo
    Conventional spin echo
    Fast spin echo
- Inversion recovery
- Gradient echo
    Coherent
    Incoherent
- Steady state free precession
- Ultra-fast imaging

This chapter serves as an introduction to pulse sequences. Further information can be found in Chapter 12.

SPIN ECHO PULSE SEQUENCES

Conventional spin echo

This pulse sequence has previously been discussed in Chapter 2. To recap, spin echo uses a 90° excitation pulse followed by one or more 180° rephasing pulses to generate a spin echo. If only one echo is generated, a T1 weighted image can be obtained using a short TE and a short TR. For proton density and T2 weighting, two RF rephasing pulses, generating two spin echoes are applied. The first echo has a short TE and a long TR to achieve proton density weighting, and the second has a long TE and a long TR to achieve T2 weighting (see Figs 2.20–2.24).

Uses

Spin echo pulse sequences are the gold standard for most imaging. They may be used for almost every examination. T1 weighted images are useful for demonstrating anatomy because they have a high SNR. In conjunction with contrast enhancement however, they can show pathology. T2 weighted images also demonstrate pathology. Tissues that are diseased are generally more oedematous and/or vascular. They have an increased water content and consequently, have a high signal on T2 weighted images and can therefore be easily identified.

Parameters

- T1 weighting
    Short TE 10–20 ms
    Short TR 300–600 ms
    Typical scan time 4–6 min
- Proton density/T2 weighting
    Short TE 20 ms/long TE 80 ms+
    Long TR 2000 ms+
    Typical scan time 7–15 min
- Advantages
    Good image quality
    Very versatile
    True T2 weighting sensitive to pathology
- Disadvantages
    Scan times relatively long

Fast spin echo

As the name suggests, fast spin echo is a spin echo pulse sequence, but with scan times that are drastically shorter than conventional spin echo.

To understand how fast spin echo achieves this, data acquisition in conventional spin echo should be re-emphasised. A 90° excitation pulse is followed by a 180° rephasing pulse. Only one phase encoding step is applied per TR on each slice and therefore, only one line of K space is filled per TR (Fig. 5.1).

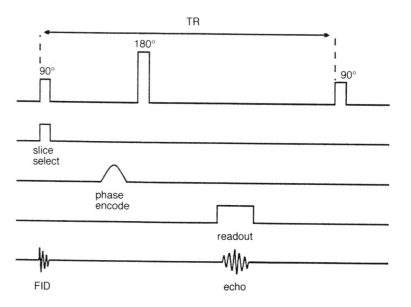

Fig. 5.1 Phase encoding in conventional spin echo.

As the scan time is a function of the TR, NEX and number of phase encodings, in order to reduce the scan time, one or more of these factors should be reduced. Decreasing the TR and the NEX affects image weighting and SNR which is undesirable. Reducing the number of phase encodings, reduces the spatial resolution which is also a disadvantage. In fast spin echo, the scan time is reduced by performing more than one phase encoding step and subsequently filling more than one line of K space per TR. This is achieved by using an echo train that consists of several 180° rephasing pulses (Fig. 5.2). At each rephasing, an echo is produced and a different phase encoding step is performed.

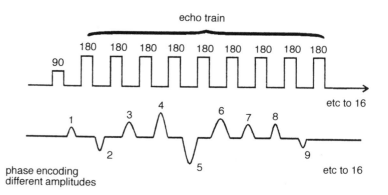

Fig. 5.2 The echo train.

In conventional spin echo, raw image data from each echo is stored in K space, and the number of 180° rephasing pulses applied corresponds to the number of echoes produced per TR. Each echo is used to produce a separate image (usually proton density and T2). In fast spin echo, data from each echo is placed into one image. The number of 180° rephasing pulses performed per TR corresponds to the number of echoes produced and the number of lines of K space filled. This number is called the *turbo factor* or the *echo train length*. The higher the turbo factor, the shorter the scan time, as more phase encoding steps are performed per TR.

For example, in conventional spin echo, 256 phase matrix selected, 256 phase encodings must be applied. Assuming 1 NEX has been selected:

256 TR times elapse to complete the scan.

In fast spin echo, using the same parameters but selecting a turbo factor of 16, 16 phase encoding steps are performed every TR. Therefore:

256/16 (16) TR times elapse to complete the scan.

The scan time is therefore reduced to a 1/16th of the original. At each 180°/phase encoding combination, a different amplitude of phase encoding gradient slope is applied in order to fill out a different line of K space. In conventional spin echo only one line is filled per TR, whereas in fast spin echo several lines corresponding to the turbo factor are filled. Therefore K space is filled more rapidly and the scan time can be reduced.

The echoes are generated at different TE times and therefore data collected from them has variable weighting. All this data is stored and

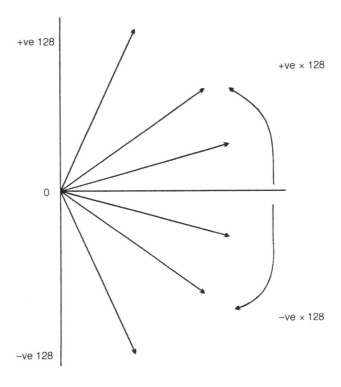

Fig. 5.3 Phase encoding gradient slopes.

placed into one image. So how is a fast spin echo sequence weighted correctly? The TE selected is only an effective TE. In other words it is the TE at which the operator wishes to weight the resultant image. In order to achieve this weighting, the system orders the phase encoding steps so that steep or shallow slopes are applied to the various echoes produced. As described in Chapter 3, each phase encoding step applies a different slope of gradient to phase shift the signal by a different amount. If 256 phase encodings are performed, the phase encoding gradient is switched on to varying degrees from +128 to −128 (Fig. 5.3).

Very steep phase encoding slopes reduce the amplitude of the resultant echo. Shallow phase encoding slopes result in an echo that has a maximum signal amplitude (Fig. 5.4).

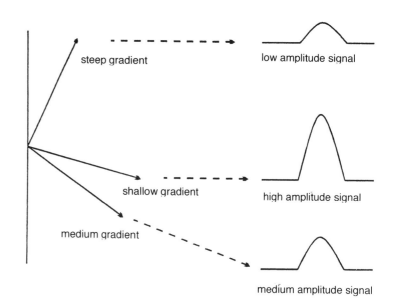

Fig. 5.4 Phase encoding slope versus signal amplitude.

The system orders the phase encodings so that the shallow slopes that produce maximum signal are centred on the effective TE selected. The steep slopes that produce a much smaller signal amplitude are placed away from the effective TE. The resultant image contains data from all the echoes in the echo train, but data from echoes collected around the effective TE has more impact on image contrast as it fills the central lines of K space which produce the greatest signal amplitude. Data from echoes collected at the wrong weighting (other TEs), has much less of an effect on the contrast, as it fills the outer lines of K space and therefore has a smaller signal amplitude and a greater spatial resolution (Fig. 5.5).

If a TE of 100 ms is selected, with a TR 3000 ms and a turbo factor of 16, T2 weighting is required. The shallowest phase encodings are performed on echoes occurring around 100 ms. Data acquired from these

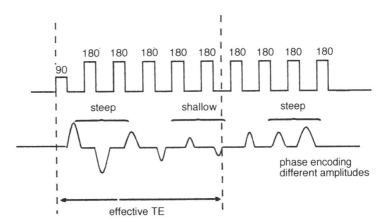

Fig. 5.5 Phase encoding ordering.

phase encodings, has a TE at or close to 100 ms. Phase encodings performed at the very beginning and end of the echo train are steep, and the signal amplitude of these echoes is small. They contain either proton density or very heavily T2 weighted data, which is present in the image but whose impact is less predominant (see Fig. 5.6).

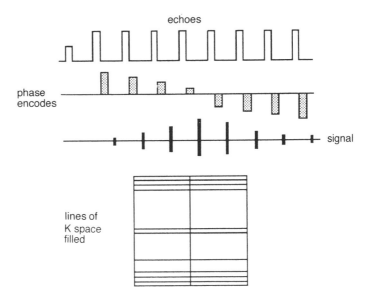

Fig. 5.6 K space filling in fast spin echo.

Uses

Generally speaking the contrast seen in fast spin echo images is similar to spin echo and, therefore, these sequences are useful in most clinical applications. In the central nervous system, pelvis and musculoskeletal regions, fast spin echo has now largely replaced spin echo. In the chest and abdomen, however, respiratory artefact is sometimes troublesome if respiratory compensation techniques are not compatible with fast spin echo software but this is offset somewhat by the fact that the shorter scan times of fast spin echo enable images with less respiratory artefact to be produced.

There are, however, two contrast differences between spin echo and fast spin echo, both of which are due to the repeated, closely spaced 180° pulses of the echo train. Firstly, fat remains bright on T2 weighted images due to the multiple RF pulses which reduce the effects of spin-spin interactions in fat (J coupling). However, fat saturation techniques can be used to compensate for this (see Chapter 6). Secondly, the repeated 180° pulses can increase magnetisation transfer effects so that muscle for example, appears darker on fast spin echo images than in conventional spin echo. In addition, the multiple 180° pulses reduce magnetic susceptibility effects which can be detrimental when looking for small haemorrhages. The plus side, however, is that artefact from metal implants is significantly reduced when using fast spin echo.

Parameters

These are similar to conventional spin echo. However, the turbo factor now plays an important role in image weighting. The higher the turbo factor, the shorter the scan time, but the resultant image has more of a mixture of weighting because there is more data collected at the wrong TE present. This is not as important in T2 weighted scans, as the proton density data is offset somewhat by the heavily T2 weighted data. In T1 and proton density weighting on the other hand, larger turbo factors place too much T2 weighting in the image and cause blurring. Image blurring occurs in fast spin echo images at the edges of tissues with different T2 decay values. This occurs because each line of K space filled during an echo train contains data from echoes with a different TE.

- Short turbo factor
  - Decreases effective TE
  - Increases T1 weighting
  - Longer scan time
  - More slices per TR
  - Reduced image blurring

- Long turbo factor
  - Increases effective TE
  - Increases T2 weighting
  - Reduces scan time
  - Reduces slice number per TR
  - Increased image blurring

The TR of fast spin echo is often much longer than those used in conventional spin echo. The 180° RF pulses take time to perform and so fewer slices are available for a given TR. As the turbo factor increases the

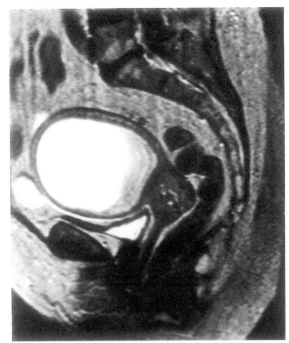

Fig. 5.7 Sagittal T2 weighted fast spin echo sequence of the pelvis, TE 102 ms, TR 4000 ms, turbo factor 16. Scan time 2 min 8 s.

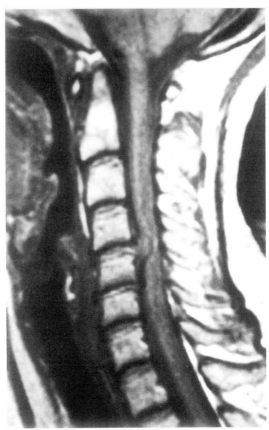

Fig. 5.8 Sagittal T1 weighted fast spin echo sequence of the cervical spine, TE 17 ms, TR 500 ms, turbo factor 4. Scan time 2 min 36 s.

number of slices available per TR decreases, and sometimes the TR has to be significantly increased in order to achieve the required slice number. In T1 weighting, increasing the TR reduces the weighting, and so in these circumstances it is probably wise to keep the TR short and to perform several acquisitions. The longer TR associated with fast spin echo somewhat offsets the reduction in scan time achieved. T1 and T2 weighted fast spin echo images are shown in Figs 5.7 and 5.8.

- T1 weighting
     Short effective TE less than 20 ms
     Short TR 300–600 ms
     Turbo factor 2–6
     Typical scan time 30 s to 1 min per acquisition

- T2 weighting
     Long effective TE 100 ms
     Long TR 4000 ms+
     Turbo factor 8–20
     Typical scan time 2 min

- Proton density/T2 weighting
     Short effective TE 20 ms/long effective TE 100 ms
     Long TR 2500 ms+
     Turbo factor 8–12
     Typical scan time 3–4 min

- Advantages
     Scan times greatly reduced
     High resolution matrices and multiple NEX can be used
     Image quality improved
     Increased T2 information

- Disadvantages
     Some flow and motion affects increased
     Incompatible with some imaging options
     Fat bright on T2 weighted images
     Image blurring can result as data is collected at different TE times
     Reduces magnetic susceptibility effect (see Chapter 7) as multiple 180° pulses produce excellent rephasing, so it should not be used when haemorrhage is suspected.

Inversion recovery

Inversion recovery is a pulse sequence that begins with a 180° inverting pulse. This inverts the NMV through 180° into full saturation. When the inverting pulse is removed, the NMV begins to relax back to B_0.

A 90° excitation pulse is then applied at a time from the 180° inverting pulse known as the *TI (time from inversion)*. The contrast of the resultant image depends primarily on the length of the TI. If the 90° excitation pulse is applied after the NMV has relaxed back through the transverse plane, the contrast in the image depends on the amount of longitudinal recovery of each vector (as in spin echo). The resultant image is heavily T1 weighted, as the 180° inverting pulse achieves full saturation and ensures a large contrast difference between fat and water (Fig. 5.9).

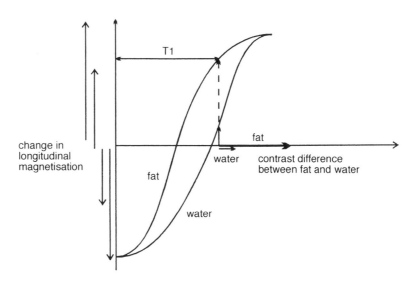

Fig. 5.9   T1 weighting in inversion recovery.

If the 90° excitation pulse is not applied until the NMV has reached full recovery, a proton density weighted image results, as both fat and water have fully relaxed (Fig. 5.10).

After the 90° excitation pulse, a 180° rephasing pulse is applied at a time TE after the excitation pulse. This produces a spin echo. The TR is the time between each 180° inverting pulse (Fig. 5.11).

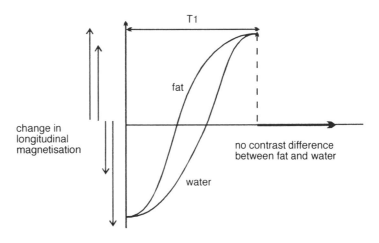

Fig. 5.10   Proton density weighting in inversion recovery.

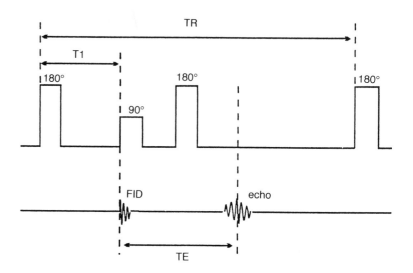

Fig. 5.11 The inversion recovery pulse sequence.

Uses

Inversion recovery was conventionally used to produce heavily T1 weighted images to demonstrate anatomy. The 180° inverting pulse produces a large contrast difference between fat and water because full saturation of the fat and water vectors is achieved at the beginning of each repetition. IR pulse sequences therefore produce more heavy T1 weighting than conventional spin echo and should be used when this is required. As the use of contrast primarily shortens the T1 times of certain tissues, IR pulse sequences increase the signal from structures that have enhanced as a result of a contrast injection. IR sequences are now more widely used in conjunction with fast spin echo to produce T2 weighted images.

Parameters

When inversion recovery is used to produce predominantly heavily T1 weighted images (Fig. 5.12), the TE controls the amount of T2 decay, and so it is usually kept short to minimise T2 effects. However, it can be lengthened to give tissues with a long T2 a bright signal. This is called pathology weighting and produces an image that is predominantly T1 weighted, but where pathological processes appear bright. The TI is the most potent controller of contrast in the inversion recovery sequence. Medium TI values give T1 weighting but, as this is lengthened, the image becomes more proton density weighted. The TR should always be long enough to allow full recovery of the NMV before the next inverting pulse is applied. If this is not so, individual vectors recover to different degrees, and the weighting is affected. To achieve full recovery of the NMV, the TR should be longer than 2000 ms. As a result the scan times are relatively long. This however is rectified on some systems which now have inversion

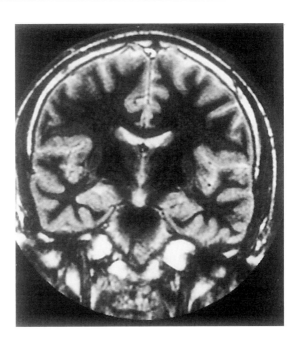

Fig. 5.12 A coronal T1 weighted inversion recovery sequence, TI 400 ms, TE 10 ms, TR 2000 ms.

recovery fast spin echo. The 180° inverting pulse is followed after the TI time by the 90° excitation pulse and the train of 180° RF pulses. This greatly reduces the scan time.

- T1 weighting
    Medium TI 400–800 ms (varies slightly at different field strengths)
    Short TE 10–20 ms
    Long TR 2000 ms+
    Average scan time 5-15 min
- Proton density weighting
    Long TI 1800 ms
    Short TE 10–20 ms
    Long TR 2000 ms+
    Average scan time 5–15 min
- Pathology weighting
    Medium TI 400–800 ms
    Long TE 70 ms+
    Long TR 2000 ms+
    Average scan time 5–15 min
- Advantages
    Very good SNR as the TR is long
    Excellent T1 contrast
- Disadvantages
    Long scan times unless used in conjunction with fast spin echo

STIR (short TI inversion recovery)

STIR is an inversion recovery pulse sequence that uses a TI that corresponds to the time it takes fat to recover from full inversion to the transverse plane so that there is no longitudinal magnetisation corresponding to fat. When the 90° excitation pulse is applied, the fat vector is flipped through 90° to 180° and into full saturation, so that the signal from fat is nulled (i.e. it gives no signal because there is no transverse component of magnetisation in fat). STIR is used to achieve suppression of the fat signal in a T1 weighted image. A TI of 100–175 ms achieves fat suppression although this value varies slightly at different field strengths. The T1 required to null the signal from a tissue is 0.69 times its T1 relaxation time. It is important to note that STIR should not be used in conjunction with contrast enhancement which shortens the T1 times of enhancing tissues thereby making them bright. The T1 times of these structures are shortened so that they approach the T1 time of fat. In a STIR sequence therefore, the enhancing tissue may also be nulled (Fig. 5.13).

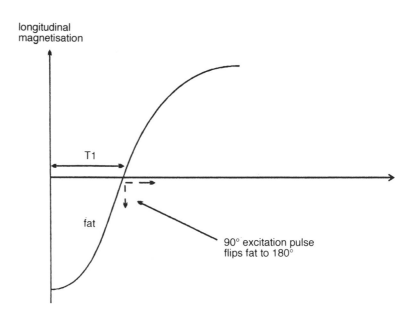

longitudinal
magnetisation

T1

fat

90° excitation pulse
flips fat to 180°

Fig. 5.13 STIR.

- Parameters
   Short TI 150–175 ms
   Short TE 10–30 ms
   Long TR 2000 ms+
   Average scan time 5–15 min

This sequence can also be used in conjunction with fast spin echo. The 180° inverting pulse is followed by a 90° excitation pulse after a short T1 and this in turn is followed by the echo train of 180° rephasing pulses as in fast spin echo. Therefore the scan time is considerably reduced compared to a conventional STIR sequence. It is mainly used with a long turbo factor and TE to produce T2 weighting with fat suppression so that the appearance of water is enhanced.

FLAIR (fluid attenuated inversion recovery)

FLAIR is another variation of the inversion recovery sequence. In FLAIR, the signal from CSF is nulled by selecting a TI corresponding to the time of recovery of CSF from 180° to the transverse plane and there is no longitudinal magnetisation present in CSF. When the 90° excitation pulse is applied, the CSF vector is flipped through 90° into full saturation again. The signal from CSF is nulled (as there is no transverse component of magnetisation in CSF), and FLAIR is used to suppress the high CSF signal in T2 and proton density weighted images so that pathology adjacent to the CSF is seen more clearly. A TI of 1700–2200 ms achieves CSF suppression (although this varies slightly at different field strengths and is calculated by multiplying the T1 relaxation time of CSF by 0.69) (Fig. 5.14).

- Parameters
    Long TI 1700–2200 ms
    Short or long TE depending on weighting required
    Long TR 6000 ms+
    Average scan time 13–20 mins

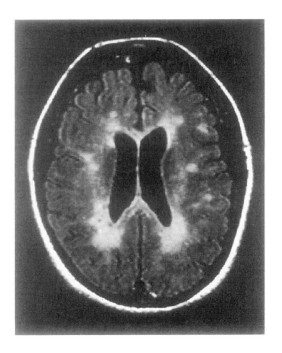

Fig. 5.14 A T2 weighted fast FLAIR image of the brain using TE 140 ms, TR 4600 ms and TI 1750 ms. The long TI has suppressed the signal from CSF improving the visualisation of the peri-ventricular MS plaques.

GRADIENT ECHO PULSE SEQUENCES

Conventional gradient echo

Gradient echo pulse sequences have been discussed in Chapter 2. To recap, gradient echo sequences use variable flip angles so that the TR and therefore the scan time, can be reduced without producing saturation. A gradient rather than a 180° rephasing RF pulse is used to rephase the FID. The frequency encoding gradient is used for this purpose because it is quicker to apply than a 180° pulse and therefore the minimum TE can be reduced. The frequency encoding gradient is initially applied negatively to speed up the dephasing of the FID, and then its polarity is reversed producing rephasing of the gradient echo. However, the gradient does not compensate for magnetic field inhomogeneities, so the resultant echo displays a great deal of $T2^*$ information (Fig. 5.15).

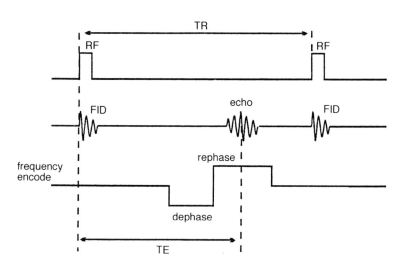

Fig. 5.15 A gradient echo pulse sequence.

Uses

Gradient echo pulse sequences can be used to acquire $T2^*$, T1, and proton density weighting. However, there is always some degree of $T2^*$ weighting present on any image due to the absence of a 180° rephasing pulse. Gradient echo sequences allow for a reduction in the scan time as the TR is greatly reduced. They can be used for single slice breath-hold acquisitions in the abdomen, and for dynamic contrast enhancement. They are very sensitive to flow as gradient rephasing is not slice selective, so flowing nuclei always give a signal, as long as they have been previously excited (see Chapter 6). Because of this, gradient echo sequences may be used to produce angiographic type images.

Parameters

The flip angle, in conjunction with the TR, determines the degree of saturation and therefore T1 weighting. To prevent saturation, the flip angles should be small and the TR long enough to permit full recovery. If saturation is required, the flip angle should be large and the TR short, so that full recovery cannot occur. The TE controls the amount of $T2^*$ dephasing. To minimise $T2^*$ the TE should be short. To maximise it, the TE should be long.

- T1 weighting
    Large flip angle 70°–110°
    Short TE 5–10 ms
    Short TR less than 50 ms
    Average scan time several seconds to minutes
- T2* weighting
    Small flip angle 5°–20°
    Long TE 15–25 ms
    Short TR full recovery as flip angle is small
    Several seconds to minutes
- Proton density weighting
    Small flip angle 5°–20°
    Short TE 5–10 ms
    Short TR full recovery as flip angle is small
    Several seconds to minutes

In conventional gradient echo the TR does not always affect image contrast. Once a certain value of TR has been exceeded, the NMV recovers fully regardless of the flip angle selected. Under these circumstances the flip angle and TE control the degree of saturation and dephasing respectively. In most systems, the conventional gradient echo sequence can be used to acquire slices in a 2D volumetric acquisition. The TR purely controls the number of slices that can be excited during the acquisition.

The steady state

The steady state is a condition where the TR is shorter than the T1 and T2 times of the tissues. There is therefore, no time for the transverse magnetisation to decay before the pulse sequence is repeated again. In the steady state, there is coexistence of both longitudinal and transverse magnetisation. The flip angle and the TR maintain the steady state which holds the longitudinal and transverse components of magnetisation and the NMV steady during the data acquisition (Fig. 5.16). Generally, flip

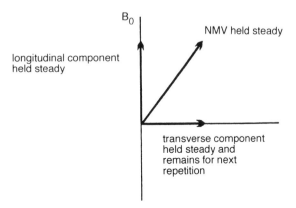

Fig. 5.16 The steady state.

angles of 30° to 45° in conjunction with a TR of 20 to 50 ms achieves the steady state.

If the steady state is maintained, the transverse component of magnetisation does not have time to decay during the pulse sequence, and therefore it affects image contrast as it induces a voltage in the receiver coil. This transverse magnetisation, produced as a result of previous excitations, is called the *residual transverse magnetisation*. It affects image contrast as it results in tissues with long T2 times (such as fluid), appearing bright on the image.

Most gradient echo sequences use the steady state as the shortest TR and scan time is achieved. Gradient echo sequences are classified according to whether the residual transverse magnetisation is in phase, (coherent), or out of phase, (incoherent). Generally, in phase residual transverse magnetisation gives tissues with a long T2 time a bright signal.

LEARNING POINT

The steady state involves repeatedly applying RF pulses at time intervals less than the T2 and T1 times of all the tissues. This train of RF pulses generates two signals;

(1) a FID signal which occurs as a result of the withdrawal of the RF pulse and contains T2* information,
(2) a spin echo whose peak occurs at the same time as an RF pulse.

This happens because every RF pulse (regardless of its net amplitude) contains individual radio waves that have sufficient energy to rephase a previous FID (Fig. 5.22). These radio waves rephase the residual transverse magnetisation left over from previous RF excitation pulses to form a spin echo. This occurs at exactly the same time as the next RF pulse as the residual transverse magnetisation takes the same time to rephase as it took to dephase in the first place (Fig. 5.17). Therefore, when utilising the steady state, the TR equals the TAU of the spin echo.

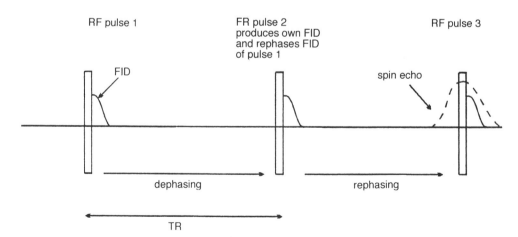

Fig. 5.17   Conditions during the steady state; a FID and a spin echo occur at each RF pulse.

To summarise – any two RF pulses produce a spin echo. The first RF pulse excites the nuclei regardless of its net amplitude, the second RF pulse rephases the FID resulting from the first RF pulse as individual radio waves within it have a magnitude of 180°. The spin echoes produced are sometimes called *Hahn* or *stimulated echoes*. This concept is re-explored later in the chapter and applies to all pulse sequences that use the steady state. At the end of the chapter, each pulse sequence will be re-evaluated with this concept in mind.

Coherent residual transverse magnetisation

Pulse sequences that use coherent magnetisation use a variable flip angle excitation pulse followed by gradient rephasing, to produce a gradient echo (Fig. 5.18). The steady state is maintained by selecting a TR shorter than the T1 and T2 times of the tissues. There is therefore residual transverse magnetisation left over when the next excitation pulse is delivered. These sequences keep this residual magnetisation coherent by a process known as *rewinding*. Rewinding is achieved by reversing the slope of the phase encoding gradient after readout. This results in the residual magnetisation rephasing, so that it is in phase at the beginning of the next repetition. This allows the residual magnetisation to build up so that tissues with a long T2 time produce a high signal.

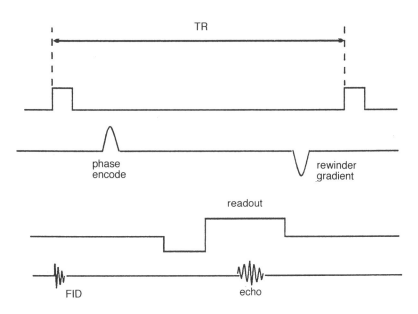

Fig. 5.18 The coherent gradient echo pulse sequence.

Uses

Coherent gradient echo pulse sequences produce images that are T2* weighted (Fig. 5.19). As fluid is bright they are often said to give an angiographic, myelographic or arthrographic effect. They can be used to

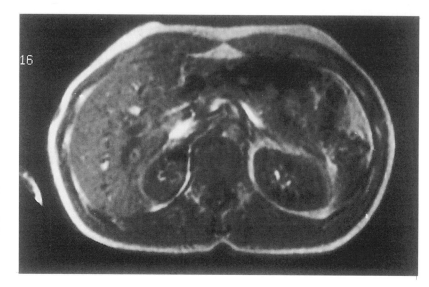

Fig. 5.19 Axial T2* weighted image of the abdomen using a coherent gradient echo pulse sequence, TE 15 ms, TR 40 ms, flip angle 35°. This image was acquired during breath-holding and took 11 s to complete.

determine whether a vessel is patent, or whether an area contains fluid. They can be acquired slice by slice, or in a 3D volume acquisition. As the TR is short, a slice can be acquired in a single breath hold.

Parameters

- To maintain the steady state
  Flip angles 30°–45°
  TR 20–50 ms
- To maximise T2*
  Long TE 15–25 ms
- Use gradient moment rephasing to accentuate T2* (see Chapter 6)
- Average scan time: seconds for single slice, 4–15 min for volumes
- (To minimise T2* to produce more T1 or proton density weighting the TE should be the shortest possible)
- Advantages
  Very fast scans, breath holding possible
  Very sensitive to flow so good for angiography
  Can be acquired in a volume acquisition
- Disadvantages
  Poor SNR in 2D acquisitions
  Magnetic susceptibility increases (see Chapter 7)
  Loud gradient noise

Incoherent (spoiled) residual transverse magnetisation

Pulse sequences that use incoherent residual transverse magnetisation, begin with a variable flip angle excitation pulse, and use gradient rephasing to produce a gradient echo. The steady state is maintained, so that residual transverse magnetisation is left over from the previous repetition. These sequences dephase or spoil this magnetisation so that its effect on image contrast is minimal. There are two ways to achieve spoiling. These are:

(1) digitised RF spoiling,
(2) gradient spoiling.

RF spoiling

RF is transmitted and received. Digitised RF can be transmitted at not only a specific frequency, but also at a specific phase. This means that the resultant NMV and transverse component of magnetisation are flipped to a certain position in the transverse plane, for example 3 o'clock. The

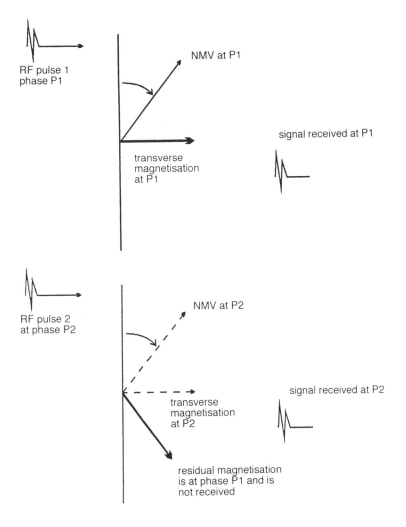

Fig. 5.20 RF spoiling.

receiver coil can lock on to the phase of the RF that has just been transmitted and receives only signal at that phase, i.e. it receives only that transverse magnetisation that was flipped to 3 o'clock. Transverse magnetisation at other phases or positions in the transverse plane are not received by the coil. This is called *RF spoiling* (Fig. 5.20) and is probably best understood with the following example.

RF pulse 1 is transmitted at phase P1 (3 o'clock)
The NMV acquires phase P1
The transverse magnetisation acquires phase P1 (i.e. it is created at position 3 o'clock on the transverse plane)
The signal received has a phase P1
RF pulse 2 is transmitted at phase P2 (9 o'clock)
The NMV acquires phase P2
The transverse magnetisation acquires phase P2 (i.e. it is created at position 9 o'clock on the transverse plane)
The signal received has a phase P2
The residual transverse magnetisation left over from RF pulse 1, is not received as it was created at 3 o'clock and the receiver coil has locked on to phase P2 (9 o'clock) and only receives signal at that phase.

This process continues for RF pulse 3, 4, etc. The residual magnetisation is ignored by the receiver coil, and its effect on image contrast is eliminated. T2* therefore cannot predominate and T1 and proton density weighting prevail.

Uses

RF spoiled pulse sequences produce T1, or proton density, weighted images, although fluid may have a rather high signal due to gradient rephasing (Fig. 5.21). They can be used for 2D and volume acquisitions, and as the TR is short the 2D acquisition can be used to acquire T1 weighted breath-hold images. RF spoiled sequences demonstrate good T1 anatomy.

Parameters

- To maintain the steady state
    Flip angle 30°–45°
    TR 20–50 ms
- To maximise T1
    Short TE 5–10 ms
- Average scan time; several seconds for single slice, 4–15 min for volumes
- Advantages
    Can be acquired in a volume or 2D
    Breath holding possible
    Good SNR and anatomical detail in volumes

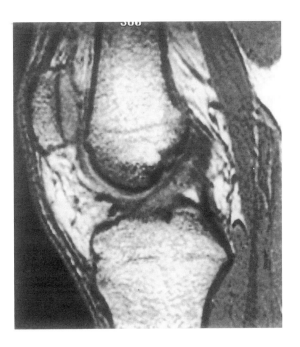

Fig. 5.21 A sagittal T1/proton density weighted image of the knee using a RF spoiling pulse sequence, TE 6 ms, TR 35 ms, flip angle 35°. This image was acquired as part of a volume acquisition which took 7 min to complete.

- Disadvantages
    SNR poor in 2D
    Loud gradient noise

Gradient spoiling

Gradients can be used to dephase as well as rephase the residual magnetisation. *Gradient spoiling* is the opposite of rewinding. In gradient spoiling, the slice select, phase encoding, and frequency encoding gradients can be used to dephase the residual magnetisation, so that it is incoherent at the beginning of the next repetition. In this way, T2* effects are reduced. Generally, the uses and parameters involved in these sequences are similar to those used in RF spoiling. However, these sequences can achieve T2* weighting when the parameters used are similar to those in conventional gradient echo. This is because gradient spoiling is less efficient than RF spoiling and so more T2* information is present in the signal.

Steady state free precession (SSFP)

SSFP can be used in the steady state so that the shortest possible TR and scan time can be achieved. However under these circumstances, the TE is never long enough to measure true T2 as a TE of 70 ms+ is required for this purpose. In addition, gradient rephasing is so inefficient that any echo is dominated by T2* effects and therefore true T2 weighting cannot be

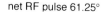

net RF pulse 61.25°

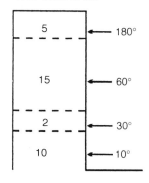

Fig. 5.22 The net effect of RF pulse energy.

achieved. Pulse sequences that employ SSFP overcome this problem to obtain images that have a sufficiently long TE and less T2* when using the steady state than other gradient echo pulse sequences. This is achieved in the following manner.

As previously described, any RF pulse contains radio waves of differing amplitudes. The magnitude of the RF pulse is merely an average of these amplitudes so that a net effect is produced. For example, an RF pulse may contain:

10 waves with amplitude of 10°,
2 with an amplitude of 30°,
15 with an amplitude of 60°,
5 with an amplitude of 180°.

The net amplitude of the RF pulse is 1960°/32 waves = 61.25° so that the RF pulse has sufficient energy to move the NMV through 61.25° (Fig. 5.22).

Therefore every RF pulse, regardless of its net magnitude, contains radio waves that on their own have sufficient magnitude to move magnetic moments within the NMV through 180°. These radio waves are therefore able to rephase a FID. In SSFP, the steady state can be maintained by using a flip angle between 30° and 45° in conjunction with a TR of 20–50 ms. Every TR an excitation pulse is applied. When the RF is switched off a FID is produced. After the TR another excitation pulse is applied which also produces its own FID. However, the radio waves within it that have an amplitude of 180° rephase the FID produced from the previous excitation pulse, and a spin echo is produced. Each RF pulse therefore not only produces its own FID, but also rephases the FID produced from the previous excitation.

As nuclei take as long to rephase as they took to dephase, the echo from the first excitation pulse occurs at the same time as the third excitation pulse (Fig. 5.23). This cannot, however, be sampled as RF

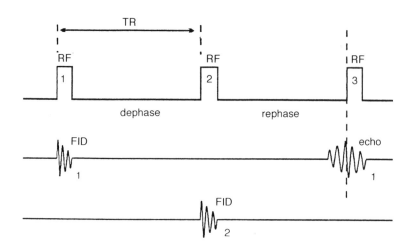

Fig. 5.23 The echo occurs at the same time as the third RF pulse.

cannot be transmitted and received at the same time. To prevent this, a rewinder gradient is used to speed up the rephasing process after the RF rephasing has begun. The rewinding moves the echo so that it occurs before the next excitation pulse, rather than during it (Fig. 5.24). In this way, the resultant echo can be received.

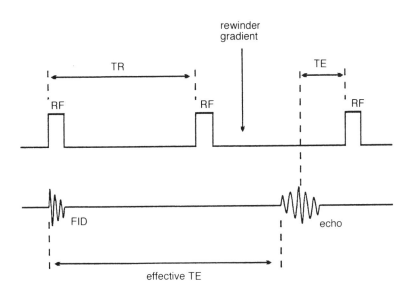

Fig. 5.24 Rewinding.

The resultant echo demonstrates more true T2 weighting than conventional gradient echo sequences. This is because:

- The TE is now longer than the TR. In SSFP, there are usually two TEs.
  (1) The actual TE is the time between the echo and the next excitation pulse.
  (2) The effective TE is the time from the echo to the excitation pulse that created its FID.
  Therefore:

$$effective\ TE = (2 \times TR) - TE$$

If the TR is 50 ms and the TE is 10 ms, then:

$$effective\ TE = (2 \times 50) - 10$$
$$= 90\ ms$$

This means that the nuclei within the echo have had 90 ms to dephase between their excitation pulse and the regeneration of the echo. T2 weighting results. Some systems rewind the echo by a set amount, for example, if the TE is fixed at 9 ms. In these circumstances:

$$effective\ TE = (2 \times TR) - 9\ ms$$

• The rephasing has been initiated by an RF pulse rather than a gradient so that more T2 and less T2* information is present. The rewinder gradient merely repositions the echo at a time when it can be received (Fig. 5.25).

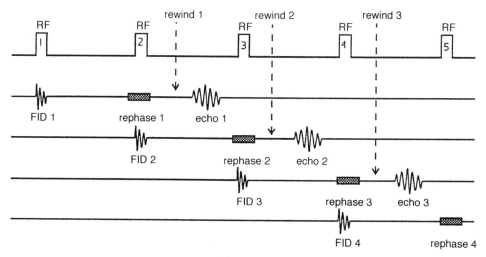

Fig. 5.25 The SSFP pulse sequence.

Uses

SSFP sequences are used to acquire images that demonstrate true T2 weighting (Fig. 5.26). They are especially useful in the brain and joints and on most systems can be used with both 2D and 3D volumetric acquisitions.

Parameters

• To maintain the steady state
    Flip angle 30°–45°
    TR 20-50 ms
• The actual TE affects the effective TE unless the system uses a fixed TE. The longer the actual TE, the lower the effective TE.
• Average scan time 4–15 min volume acquisition
• Some manufacturers suggest decreasing the effective TE to reduce magnetic susceptibility, and increasing the flip angle to create more transverse magnetisation which results in higher SNR.
• Advantages
    Can be acquired in a volume and in 2D
    True T2 weighting achieved
• Disadvantages
    Susceptible to artefacts
    Image quality can be poor
    Loud gradient noise

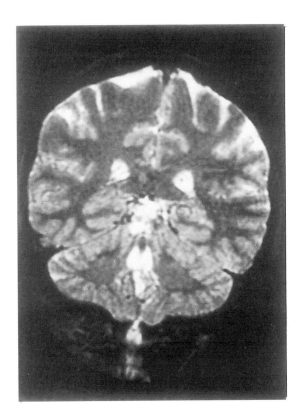

Fig. 5.26 A coronal SSFP image of the brain, effective TE 71 ms, TE 9 ms, TR 40 ms, flip angle 35°. This image was acquired as part of a volume acquisition and took 9 min to complete.

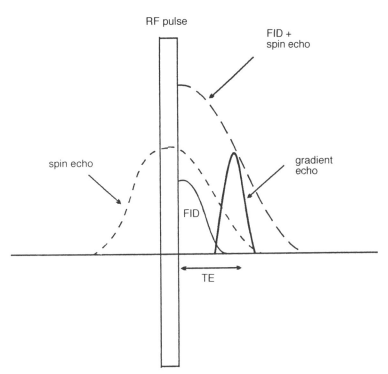

Fig. 5.27 Conditions during a coherent gradient echo pulse sequence.

LEARNING POINT

As previously explained, the steady state produces two signals:

(1) a FID,
(2) a spin echo made up of the residual transverse magnetisation component.

Coherent, incoherent and SSFP pulse sequences can be differentiated according to whether they use one, or both of these signals.

Coherent pulse sequences use a gradient to rephase both the FID and the dephasing portion of the spin echo (Fig. 5.27).

Incoherent pulse sequences use a gradient to rephase the FID only. The spin echo which contains the residual transverse magnetisation is spoiled by RF or gradient spoiling and is not sampled (Fig. 5.28).

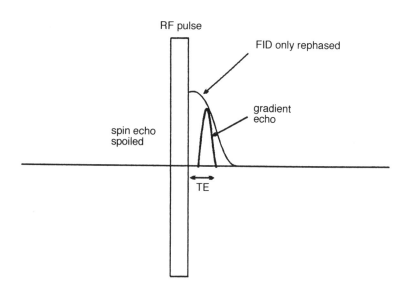

Fig. 5.28 Conditions during an incoherent gradient echo sequence.

SSFP uses an RF pulse to initiate the rephasing process, and a rewinder to move the spin echo so that it occurs before the RF pulse. The FID is not rephased and is not sampled. It only serves as a future source of residual transverse magnetisation that will form a spin echo two repetitions later (Fig. 5.29).

Ultra-fast sequences

The most recent advances have been made in developing very fast pulse sequences that can acquire several slices in a single breath hold. These usually employ the coherent or incoherent gradient echo sequences but the TE is significantly reduced. This is achieved by applying only a portion of the RF excitation pulse, so that it takes much less time to apply and switch off. In addition, only a proportion of the echo is read (partial echo). These measures ensure that the TE is kept to a minimum (2.5–3.0 ms), so that the TR and therefore the scan time can be reduced accordingly. A TR

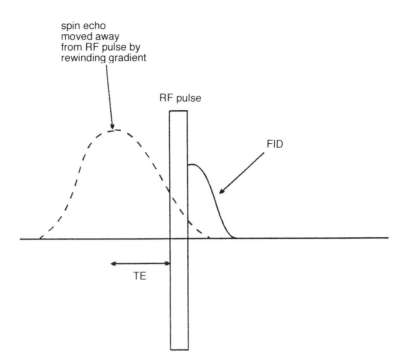

spin echo
moved away
from RF pulse by
rewinding gradient

RF pulse

FID

TE

Fig. 5.29 Conditions during a
steady state free precession
sequence.

as low as 10 ms can be achieved in this manner and this enables up to
about 16 slices to be acquired in a single breath hold. In addition, many
ultra-fast sequences use extra pulses applied before the pulse sequence
begins, to pre-magnetise the tissue. In this way, certain contrast can be
obtained. To date, this pre-magnetisation is achieved in the following two
ways.

(1) A 180° pulse is applied before the pulse sequence begins. This inverts
the NMV into full saturation and at a specified delay time, the pulse
sequence itself begins. This can be used to null signal from certain
organs and tissues and is similar to inversion recovery.
(2) A 90°/180°/90° combination is applied before the pulse sequence
begins. The first 90° pulse produces transverse magnetisation. The
180° pulse rephases this, and at a specified time later the second 90°
pulse is applied. This drives the coherent transverse magnetisation
into the longitudinal plane, so that it is available to be flipped when the
pulse sequence begins. This is used to produce T2 contrast and is
sometimes known as *driven equilibrium*.

K space filling and weighting

Weighting is achieved in these sequences by applying all the shallowest
phase encoding gradients first, and leaving the steep ones until the end of
the pulse sequence. In this way, the effect of the pre-magnetisation

prevails, as when it is dominant the central phase encodings (that produce the greatest signal amplitudes and determine the weighting of the sequence) are performed. By the end of the sequence, the pre-magnetisation has decayed and this is when the low signal amplitudes are acquired.

Echo planar imaging (EPI)

As shown in fast spin echo, the scan time is significantly reduced by filling more than one line of K space at once. Taking this concept to the limits, the fastest scan time possible would be one where all the lines are filled after one repetition. This forms the basis of EPI. EPI is an MR acquisition method that collects all the data required to fill all the lines of K space from a single echo train. In order to achieve this multiple echoes are generated and each is phase encoded by a different slope of gradient to fill all the required lines of K space. For example, if a phase matrix of 128 is required then an echo train of 128 echoes is produced and individually phase encoded to fill 128 lines of K space. Echoes are generated either by 180° rephasing pulses (termed spin echo EPI), or by gradients (termed gradient echo EPI). If RF pulses are exclusively utilised for this purpose then the RF deposition to the patient would probably exceed safety limits and the echo train would take so long to perform that most of the signal would be lost before a satisfactory amount of data could be acquired. Gradient rephasing, however, is much faster and involves no RF deposition to the patient but does require high speed gradients. In order to fill all of K space in one repetition, the readout and phase encode gradients must rapidly switch on and off. To understand why this is necessary, a review of K space traversal in conventional spin echo sequences is required.

In conventional spin echo, one line of K space is filled every TR. The position of this line depends upon the amplitude and polarity of the phase gradient. The amplitude and polarity of the readout gradient does not change and therefore each line is filled in the same direction (usually from left to right). A nice way of understanding this is to imagine that you are drawing the lines of K space with a pen as they are filled. During conventional imaging, every TR the pen is placed on the left-hand side of K space and moved across the page to the right-hand side during data acquisition. During the next TR period, when another line of K space is filled, the pen must be lifted off the paper and placed on the left-hand margin of K space again to begin the next line. This process is repeated every TR interval (Fig. 5.30).

In EPI all of K space is filled after a single repetition, i.e. there is no TR. Only one excitation pulse is applied and, from this, data to fill all of K space is acquired. In the example shown in Fig. 5.31, which is termed snapshot EPI, all of the lines are filled *without removing the pen from the paper*. There are several ways of achieving this – the simplest version is described here.

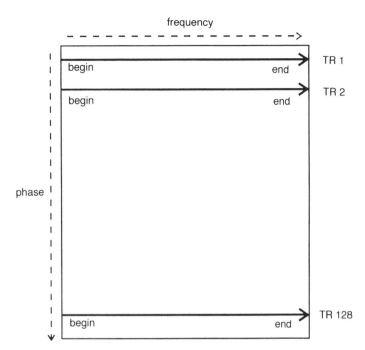

Fig. 5.30 K space filling in conventional spin echo. One line of K space is filled per TR.

As discussed in Chapter 3, K space traversal is dictated by the amplitude and polarity of both the readout and phase gradients. To recap:

- *frequency* encoding gradient *positive*, K space traversed *from left to right*
- *frequency* encoding gradient *negative*, K space traversed *from right to left*

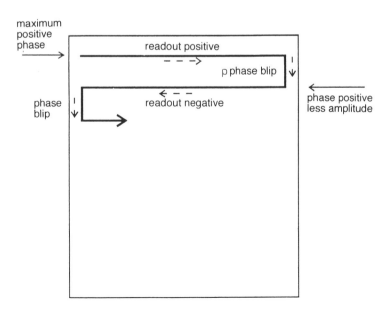

Fig. 5.31 Oscillation of frequency, blipping of phase.

- *phase* encoding gradient *positive*, fills *top* half of K space
- *phase* encoding gradient *negative*, fills *bottom* half of K space

Filling K space in EPI involves rapidly switching the readout gradient from positive to negative; positively to fill a line of K space from left to right and negatively to fill a line from right to left. This rapid change in gradient polarity also rephases the FID produced after the excitation pulse to generate the echoes within the echo train. As the readout gradient switches its polarity so rapidly it is said to oscillate.

The phase gradient also has to switch on and off rapidly but its polarity does not need to change in this type of K space traversal. The first application of the phase gradient is maximum positive to fill the top line. The next application (to encode the next echo in the echo train) is still positive but its amplitude is slightly less so that the next line down is filled. This process is repeated until the centre of K space is reached when the phase gradient switches negatively to fill the bottom lines. The amplitude is gradually increased until maximum negative polarity is achieved filling the bottom line of K space. This type of gradient switching is called blipping (Fig. 5.31).

A more complex type of K space traversal is shown in Fig. 5.32. In this example both the readout and the phase gradient switch their polarity rapidly and oscillate. In this spiral form of K space traversal, not only does the readout gradient oscillate to fill lines from left to right and then right to left, but as K space filling begins at the centre, the phase gradient must also oscillate to fill a line in the top half followed by a line in the bottom half. To understand this more clearly, place a pen at the centre of K space on the diagram and work out the amplitude and polarity of each gradient as you move your pen along. In this example, the pen is never removed

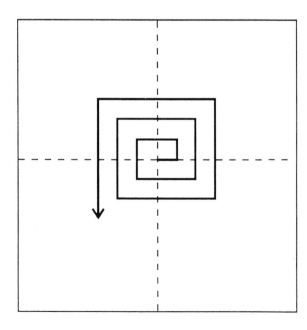

Fig. 5.32 Spiral K space traversal in EPI.

from the paper indicating that there is no TR; all of K space is filled in one go.

As data acquisition is so rapid in EPI, images may be acquired in 50–80 ms. Axial images of the whole brain are possible in 2–3 s and whole body imaging in about 30 s. There are drawbacks however. EPI sequences place exceptional strains on the gradients and therefore gradient modifications are required at significant cost. The slew rates of the gradients must be about 4 times that of conventional gradients (see Chapter 12). Two types of gradient power supply modifications can be utilised:

- *Resonant* power supplies allow the readout and phase gradients to oscillate at the same frequency thereby reducing gradient requirements. The disadvantage is that they are only able to operate at a fixed frequency and amplitude. In practical terms this means that the gradients could only be used for EPI sequences so that the system would require two power supplies; one for EPI and one for conventional imaging.
- *Non-resonant* power supplies produce any gradient waveform so that both EPI and conventional sequences may be run off the same supply. This significantly reduces the cost but also the specifications of the gradients as they have to be able to cope with both types of sequence.

Contrast and artefacts

Some typical pulse sequence diagrams for EPI are shown in Figs 5.33 and 5.34. As all of K space is filled at once, the recovery rates of individual tissues are not critical. For this reason the TR is said to equal infinity (because it is infinitely long). Either proton density or T2 weighting is achieved by selecting either a short or long effective TE which corresponds to the time interval between the excitation pulse and when the centre of K space is filled. T1 weighting is possible by applying an inverting pulse prior to the excitation pulse to produce saturation.

Typical parameters

EPI images are plagued with artefacts. As all the echoes must be encoded before the transverse magnetisation has decayed to zero, images contain a significant amount of T2* decay. This is not compensated for by gradient rephasing. In addition, SNR in the snapshot version of EPI is relatively poor. To compensate for these effects several modifications to the basic EPI sequence have been made. Firstly, *hybrid* sequences which integrate fast spin echo and EPI, have been developed. These sequences combine both gradient and RF pulses to generate the echoes in the echo train. Typically a series of gradient rephasings are followed by an RF rephasing pulse. The hybrid sequence utilises the benefits of both types of

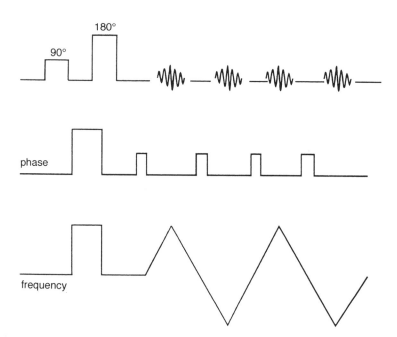

Fig. 5.33   Spin echo EPI.

rephasing methods; the speed of the gradient *and* the ability of the RF pulse to compensate for T2* effects. These sequences increase the scan time to over 100 ms per image but the benefits in terms of image quality are significant.

In addition, SNR is improved by acquiring only a portion of K space at a time. There are two ways of achieving this:

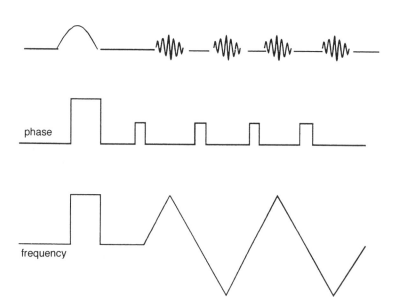

Fig. 5.34   Gradient echo EPI

(1) *K space segmentation by acquisition* acquires a quarter of K space at a time so that there are four excitations and TR periods. If a 128 phase matrix is required then a turbo factor of 32, repeated four times, fills K space.

(2) *K space segmentation by echo* utilises a turbo factor of four that is repeated 32 times. Data from the first echoes is placed in the top quarter of K space, data from the second echoes in the next quarter and so on.

Both methods increase the scan time by a factor of four but produce images with improved quality when compared with snapshot acquisitions.

Another problem with EPI is that fat signal is misregistered. Fat saturation techniques are therefore commonly required to compensate.

Uses and limitations

EPI has a huge potential to revolutionise clinical MRI. Rapid data acquisition has enabled the development of real-time MRI which forms the basis of the new interventional system from General Electric. MR therapy using real-time data acquisition is still under review but the advantages of safety, three dimensionality and the sensitivity of the MR signal to temperature changes resulting from cryotherapy will almost certainly result in an increase in the application of this technology (see Chapter 12).

Rapid image acquisition is also ideal for functional imaging where changes in blood oxygenation in response to cortical function result in a rapid alteration of the MR signal which can be measured using EPI. The potential applications of this modality are astounding. Apart from increasing our knowledge of brain function, this technology is useful to map out areas of crucial function prior to surgery and to investigate how certain tasks may be re-learned following brain injury (see Chapter 12).

EPI will almost certainly increase the use of MR in the chest and abdomen as data acquisition is so rapid physiological motion is frozen. Detailed imaging of the heart and coronary vessels are possible using EPI. The speed and quality of abdominal imaging will also improve thereby increasing MR applications in these areas.

Concerns over safety have, however, been expressed. The rapid switching of gradients causes nerve stimulation and gradient noise is severe and acoustic insulation and ear protection are essential. Despite these problems EPI and hybrid sequences will almost certainly replace more conventional sequences in the future.

Summary

The choice of each pulse sequence is often a quite difficult one. There are now so many available that we are really spoilt for choice. However, generally speaking every pulse sequence is designed to produce a certain

Table 5.1 A comparison of the acronyms used by manufacturers.

	GE	Philips	Siemens	Picker	Elscint	Hitachi	Shimadzu
Spin echo	MEMP VEMP	spin echo	spin echo	spin echo	spin echo	spin echo	spin echo
Fast spin echo	FSE	TSE	TSE	FSE		FSE	
Coherent gradient echo	GRASS	FFE	FISP	FAST	F short	GFEC	SSFP
Incoherent gradient echo (RF spoiled)	SPGR	T1 FFE		RF spoiled FAST			STAGE T1W
Incoherent gradient echo (gradient spoiled)	MPGR		FLASH		short	GRE	STAGE
Steady state free precession	SSFP	T2 FFE	PSIF	CE FAST	E short	GFEC contrast	STERF
Inversion recovery	MPIR	IR	IR	IR	IR	IR	IR
Short T1 inversion recovery	STIR	SPIR	STIR	STIR	STIR	STIR	STIR
Ultra fast	fast GRASS SPGR (IR/DE prep)	TFE	Turbo FLASH 3D MP RAGE	RAM FAST			SMASH
Pre-saturation	SAT	REST	SAT	pre-SAT	spatial pre-sat	SAT	SAT
Gradient moment rephasing	flow comp	FLAG	GMR	MAST	STILL	GR	SMART
Resp. compensation	resp. comp	PEAR	resp. trigger	resp. gating PRIZE	FREEZE	phase re-ordering	
Signal averaging	NEX	NSA	AC	NSA		NSA	
Partial averaging	fractional NEX	half scan	half Fourier	phase conjugate symmetry	single side encoding	half Fourier	
Partial echo	fractional echo	partial echo		read conjugate symmetry	single side view		
No phase wrap	no phase wrap	fold over suppression	over sampling	over sampling	anti aliasing	anti wrap	
Rectangular FOV	rect FOV	rect FOV	half Fourier imaging	under sampling	rect FOV	rect FOV	

Abbreviations used in Table 5.1.

3D MP RAGE	3D magnetisation prepared rapid gradient echo
AC	Number of acquisitions
CE FAST	Contrast enhanced FAST
DE prep	Driven equilibrium magnetisation preparation
E short	Short repetition technique based on echo
FAST	Fourier acquired steady state technique
FFE	Fast field echo
FISP	Fast imaging with steady precession
FLAG	Flow adjusted gradients
FLASH	Fast low angled shot
FREEZE	Respiratory selection of phase encoding steps
FSE	Fast spin echo
F short	Short repetition technique based on free induction decay
GFE	Gradient field echo
GFEC	Gradient field echo with contrast
GMR	Gradient moment rephasing
GR	Gradient rephasing
GRASS	Gradient recalled acquisition in the steady state
IR prep	Inversion recovery magnetisation preparation
MAST	Motion artefact suppression

MEMP	Multi echo multi planar
MPGR	Multi planar gradient recalled acquisition in the steady state
MPIR	Multi planar inversion recovery
NEX	Number of excitations
NSA	Number of signal averages
PEAR	Phase encoding artefact reduction
PSIF	Mirrored FISP
RAM FAST	Rapid acquisition matrix FAST
REST	Regional saturation technique
RF spoiled FAST	RF spoiled Fourier acquired steady state
Short	Short repetition techniques
SMART	Shimadzu motion artefact reduction technique
SMASH	Short minimum angled shot
SPGR	Spoiled gradient recalled acquisition in the steady state
SPIR	Spectrally selective inversion recovery
SSFP	Steady state free precession
STAGE	Small tip angle gradient echo
STERF	Steady state technique with refocused FID
STILL	Flow motion compensation
STIR	Short TI inversion recovery
TFE	Turbo field echo
TSE	Turbo spin echo
Turbo FLASH	Magnetisation prepared sub second imaging technique
VEMP	Variable echo multi planar

contrast, image quality and data acquisition. These factors should be taken into account when selecting a particular pulse sequence. Table 5.1 should help most readers apply the terms used in this, and other chapters to their type of system.

Questions

1. Which pulse sequence would you choose for each of the following and why?
   (a) T1 weighted breath hold
   (b) Steady state T2*
   (c) True T2 weighted volume.

2. Explain why RF spoiled pulse sequences are not the best choice when T2* weighting is required.

3. Explain why SSFP is not the best choice when a T1 weighted image is required.

4. List the differences between spin echo and gradient echo sequences.

5. What are the effects of lengthening the turbo factor in fast spin echo?

6. Match the following relationships:

   In coherent gradient echo   only the spin echo are sampled
   In incoherent gradient echo   the FID and the spin echo are sampled
   In SSFP   only the FID is sampled.

7. In resonant gradient systems:
   (a) the frequency and phase gradients oscillate
   (b) the frequency gradient oscillates, the phase gradient blips
   (c) gradients transmit RF at the Larmor frequency.

Chapter 6   Flow Phenomena

Introduction

This chapter specifically explores artefacts produced from nuclei that move during the acquisition of data. Flowing nuclei exhibit different contrast characteristics from their neighbouring stationary nuclei, and originate primarily from nuclei in blood and CSF. The motion of flowing nuclei causes mismapping of signals and results in artefacts known as flow motion artefacts or phase ghosting. The causes of flow artefact are collectively known as *flow phenomena*. The principal phenomena are:

(1) time of flight,
(2) entry slice phenomenon,
(3) intra-voxel dephasing.

First however, the common mechanisms and types of flow are analysed.

The mechanisms of flow

There are four principal types of flow (Fig. 6.1):

(1) *Laminar flow* is flow that is at different but consistent velocities across a vessel. The flow at the centre of the lumen of the vessel is faster than at the vessel wall, where resistance slows down the flow. However, the velocity difference across the vessel is constant.
(2) *Turbulent flow* is flow at different velocities that fluctuates randomly. The velocity difference across the vessel changes erratically.
(3) *Vortex flow* is flow that is initially laminar but then passes through a stricture or stenosis in the vessel. Flow in the centre of the lumen has a high velocity but near the walls, the flow spirals.

(4) *Stagnant flow* is where the velocity of flow slows to a point of stagnation. The signal intensity of stagnant flow depends on its T1, T2 and proton density characteristics. In other words, it behaves like stationary tissue.

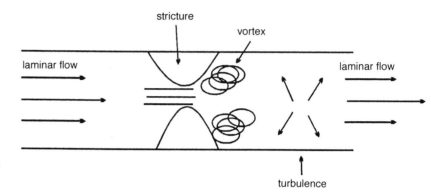

Fig. 6.1 The different types of flow.

LEARNING POINT

Flow mechanisms are often termed as follows:

First order motion   laminar flow (constant velocity)
Second order motion   acceleration
Third order motion   jerk

At present only first order flow can be compensated for.

Time of flight phenomenon

In order to produce a signal, a nucleus must receive an excitation pulse and a rephasing pulse. If a nucleus receives the excitation pulse only and is not rephased, it does not produce a signal. Similarly, if a nucleus is rephased but has not previously been excited, it does not produce a signal. Stationary nuclei always receive both excitation and rephasing pulses, but flowing nuclei present in the slice for the excitation may have exited the slice before rephasing. This is called *time of flight phenomenon* (Fig. 6.2). The effects of the time of flight phenomenon depend on the type of pulse sequence used.

Time of flight in spin echo pulse sequences

In a spin echo pulse sequence, a 90° excitation pulse and a 180° rephasing pulse are applied to each slice. Every slice is therefore selectively excited and rephased. Stationary nuclei within the slice receive both the 90° and the 180° RF pulses and produce a signal.

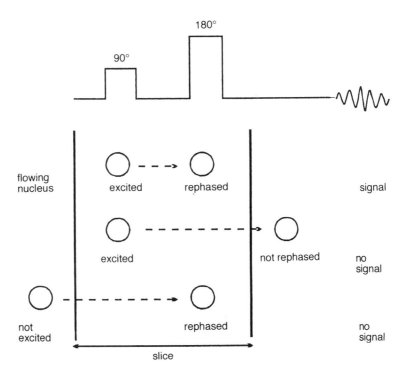

Fig. 6.2 The time of flight phenomenon.

Nuclei flowing perpendicular to the slices may be present within the slice during the 90° pulse, but may have exited the slice before the 180° pulse can be delivered. These nuclei are excited but not rephased and do not therefore give a signal. Alternatively nuclei not present in the slice during excitation may be present during rephasing. These nuclei have not previously been excited and do not therefore give a signal. Time of flight phenomena result in a signal void from the nuclei; and so the vessel appears dark. Time of flight effects depend on the:

(1) velocity of flow,
(2) TE,
(3) slice thickness.

Velocity of flow

As the velocity of flow increases, a smaller proportion of flowing nuclei are present in the slice for both the 90° and the 180° RF pulses. As the velocity of flow increases, the time of flight effect increases. This is called *high velocity signal loss*.

As the velocity of flow decreases, a higher proportion of flowing nuclei are present in the slice for both the 90° and the 180° RF pulses. Therefore as the velocity of flow decreases, the time of flight effect decreases. This is called *flow related enhancement*.

The TE

As the TE increases, a higher proportion of flowing nuclei have exited the slice between the excitation pulse and the 180° rephasing pulse. Therefore, at a longer TE, more nuclei have received only one pulse and the signal void increases (Fig. 6.3).

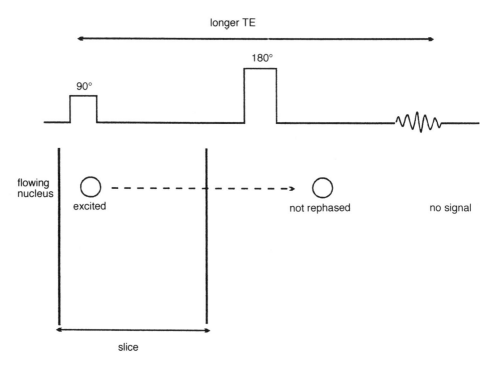

Fig. 6.3   Time of flight versus TE.

Slice thickness

For a given constant velocity, nuclei take longer to travel through a thick slice compared with a thin slice. Therefore, nuclei are more likely to receive both the 90° and 180° pulse in thick slices. As the thickness of the slice decreases, the nuclei are more likely to receive only one pulse and the signal void increases.

Time of flight in gradient echo pulse sequences

In gradient echo pulse sequences a variable excitation pulse is followed by gradient rephasing. Each slice is selectively excited by the RF pulse but the rephasing gradient is applied to the whole body. In other words, the excitation pulse is slice selective, but the gradient rephasing is not.

Therefore, a flowing nucleus that receives an excitation pulse is rephased regardless of its slice position and produces a signal. In addition, the very short TR usually associated with gradient echo sequences, tends to saturate stationary nuclei which receive repeated RF pulses so that flowing nuclei appear to have a higher signal. This is explored later. In gradient echo pulse sequences therefore, flow signal enhancement is increased and these pulse sequences are often said to be flow sensitive.

- Time of flight phenomena produce flow related enhancement or high velocity signal loss.
- Flow related enhancement increases as the:
    velocity of flow decreases
    TE decreases,
    slice thickness increases.
- High velocity signal void increases as the:
    velocity of flow increases,
    TE increases,
    slice thickness decreases.

Entry slice phenomenon (in-flow effect)

Entry slice phenomenon is related to the excitation history of the nuclei. Nuclei that receive repeated RF pulses during the acquisition are said to be saturated or 'beaten down'. The NMV of these nuclei eventually reach an equilibrium position, and produce a signal according to the TE, TR, flip angle and contrast characteristics of the tissue in which the protons are situated.

Nuclei that have not received these repeated RF pulses are said to be 'fresh', as their NMV has not been beaten down by successive RF pulses. The signal that they produce is different from that of the saturated nuclei (Fig. 6.4).

Stationary nuclei within a slice become saturated after repeated RF pulses. Nuclei flowing perpendicular to the slice enter the slice fresh, as they were not present during repeated excitations. They therefore produce a different signal from the stationary nuclei. This is called *entry slice phenomenon* or in-flow effect as it is most prominent in the first slice of a 'stack' of slices.

The slices in the middle of the stack exhibit less entry slice phenomenon, as flowing nuclei have received more excitation pulses by the time they reach these slices. In other words, they become less fresh and more saturated and their signal intensity depends mostly on the TE, TR, flip angle and the contrast characteristics of the tissue in which they are situated.

Entry slice phenomena only decrease if nuclei receive repeated excitations. The rate at which the nuclei receive the excitation pulses determines the magnitude of the phenomenon. Any factor that affects the rate at which a nucleus receives repeated excitations affects the magnitude

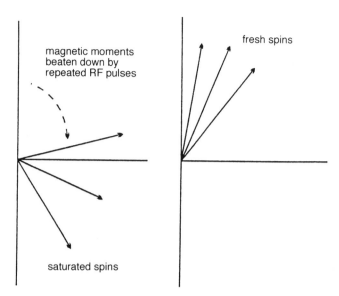

fresh spins

magnetic moments
beaten down by
repeated RF pulses

Fig. 6.4 Contrast differences
between saturated and fresh
spins.

saturated spins

of the phenomenon. The magnitude of entry slice phenomenon therefore
depends on:

(1) TR,
(2) slice thickness,
(3) velocity of flow,
(4) direction of flow.

The TR is the time between each excitation pulse. A short TR results in an
increase in the rate at which the RF is delivered. In other words a short TR
decreases the time between successive RF pulses. A short TR therefore
reduces the magnitude of entry slice phenomena.

Flowing nuclei with a constant velocity take longer to travel through
thick slices than thin slices. Nuclei travelling through thick slices are likely
to receive more RF pulses than nuclei travelling through thin slices. Entry
slice phenomenon therefore increases in thick slices compared with thin
slices.

The velocity of flow also affects the rate at which a flowing nucleus
receives RF. Fast flowing nuclei are more likely to have travelled to the
next slice when RF is delivered than slow nuclei. Entry slice phenomenon
is therefore increased as the velocity of flow increases.

The direction of flow is probably the most important factor in
determining the magnitude of entry slice phenomenon. Flow that is in
the same direction as slice selection is called co-current. Flow that is in the
opposite direction to slice selection is called counter-current flow.

Co-current flow

Flowing nuclei travel in the same direction as slice selection. The flowing
nuclei are more likely to receive repeated RF excitations as they move

from one slice to the next. They therefore become saturated relatively quickly, and so entry slice phenomenon decreases rapidly.

Counter-current flow

Flowing nuclei travel in the opposite direction to slice excitation. Flowing nuclei stay fresh as when they enter a slice they are less likely to have received previous excitation pulses. Entry slice phenomenon does not therefore decrease rapidly and may still be present deep within the slice stack (Fig. 6.5).

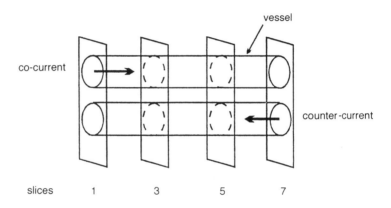

Fig. 6.5 Co- and counter-current flow.

- Entry slice phenomenon increases:
  at the first slice in the stack,
  when using a long TR,
  in thin slices,
  with fast flow,
  in counter-current flow.

Intra-voxel dephasing

Gradients alter the magnetic field strength, precessional frequency and phase of nuclei. Nuclei flowing along a gradient rapidly accelerate or decelerate depending on the direction of flow and gradient application. Flowing nuclei therefore either gain phase (if they have been accelerated), or lose phase (if they have been decelerated).

If a flowing nucleus is adjacent to a stationary nucleus in a voxel, there is a phase difference between the two nuclei. This is because the flowing nucleus has either lost or gained phase relative to the stationary nucleus due to its motion along the gradient. Therefore nuclei within the same voxel are out of phase with each other, which results in a reduction of total signal amplitude from the voxel. This is called *intra-voxel dephasing* (Fig. 6.6). The magnitude of intra-voxel dephasing depends on the degree

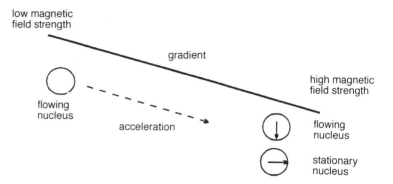

Fig. 6.6 Intra-voxel dephasing.

of turbulence. In turbulent flow, intra-voxel dephasing effects are irreversible. In laminar flow, the intra-voxel dephasing can be compensated for as long as the velocity of flow is constant.

- Flow affects image quality.
- Time of flight effects give signal void or enhancement.
- Entry slice phenomenon effects give a different signal intensity to flowing nuclei.
- The signal intensity of the lumen is also affected by the mechanism of flow.

FLOW PHENOMENA COMPENSATION

Introduction

Flowing nuclei therefore produce a very confusing range of signal intensities. Ideally, these should be compensated for, so that their adverse effects on image quality and interpretation can be minimised. There are several methods available to help reduce flow artefacts and these are now discussed.

Gradient moment rephasing (nulling)

Gradient moment rephasing compensates for the altered phase values of the nuclei flowing along a gradient. It uses additional gradients to correct the altered phases back to their original values. In this way, flowing nuclei do not gain or lose phase due to the presence of the main gradient.

Gradient moment rephasing is performed by the slice select gradient and/or the readout gradient. The gradient alters its polarity from positive to double negative and then back to positive again. A flowing nucleus travelling along these gradients, experiences different magnetic field strengths. Therefore its precessional frequency changes accordingly.

In order to compensate altered phase values, the precessional frequency at the beginning of gradient moment rephasing must be the same as it is at the end. The net precessional frequency and phase change must therefore be zero (Fig. 6.7).

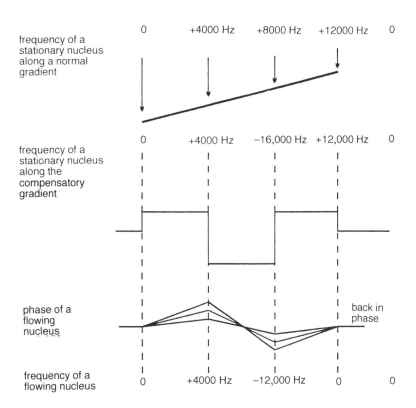

Fig. 6.7 Gradient moment rephasing (nulling).

Let us assume the gradient changes the precessional frequency by 4000 Hz per cm. At 1 cm along the gradient the precessional frequency will be 4000 Hz, at 2 cm 8000 Hz, and at 3 cm 12000 Hz. Let us also assume, for easy mathematics, that the precessional frequency at the beginning of the gradient is zero, (of course in practice it is approximately the Larmor frequency). In order to compensate properly, the precessional frequency of a nucleus flowing along the gradient must be zero by the time it gets to the end of the gradient. In this way, the net phase change of a flowing nucleus will also be zero.

The positive portion of the compensatory gradient changes the precessional frequency of a flowing nucleus from zero to +4000 Hz.

The double negative gradient is then applied. On its own, it would alter the precessional frequency to −16000 Hz (to −8000 × 2 as gradient amplitude is doubled). However, the flowing nucleus previously had a precessional frequency of +4000 Hz, so the net frequency change of the flowing nucleus is −12000 Hz.

The positive gradient is then reapplied. On its own, this gradient would alter the precessional frequency from +8000 Hz to +12000 Hz. As the flowing nucleus previously had a precessional frequency of −12000 Hz, the net change is zero (–12 000 to +12 000). As the net precessional frequency change is zero, the phase change of the flowing nucleus is also zero.

Gradient moment rephasing reduces intra-voxel dephasing. As flowing nuclei have the same phase as stationary nuclei in the same voxel, their signals add constructively and therefore a bright signal results. Gradient moment rephasing gives flowing nuclei a bright signal as spins are in phase. Figure 6.8 shows axial gradient echo images of the abdomen with and without gradient moment rephasing.

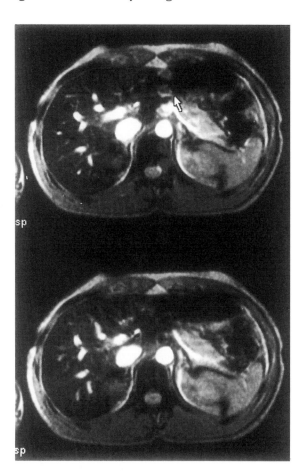

Fig. 6.8 Axial gradient echo images of the abdomen. The upper image shows mismapping of the flowing nuclei within the aorta (arrow). The lower image uses gradient moment rephasing to compensate for this.

Gradient moment rephasing assumes a constant velocity across the gradients at all times. It is most effective on slow laminar flow and is therefore often termed first order motion compensation. Pulsatile flow is not strictly constant so gradient moment rephasing is often more effective on venous rather than arterial flow. It is also less effective on turbulent, fast flow perpendicular to the slice. As gradient moment rephasing uses extra gradients, it increases the minimum TE. If the system has to perform extra gradient tasks, more time must elapse before it is ready to read an echo. As a result, fewer slices may be available for a given TR. As flowing nuclei are bright when gradient moment rephasing is selected, it is usually used in T2 and T2* weighted sequences where fluid (blood and CSF) is bright anyway.

Pre-saturation

Pre-saturation pulses nullify the signal from flowing nuclei so that the effects of entry slice and time of flight phenomena are minimised. Pre-saturation delivers a 90° RF pulse to a volume of tissue outside the FOV. A flowing nucleus within the volume receives this 90° pulse. When it then enters the slice stack, it receives an excitation pulse and is saturated. If it is fully saturated to 180°, it has no transverse component of magnetisation and produces a signal void (Fig. 6.9).

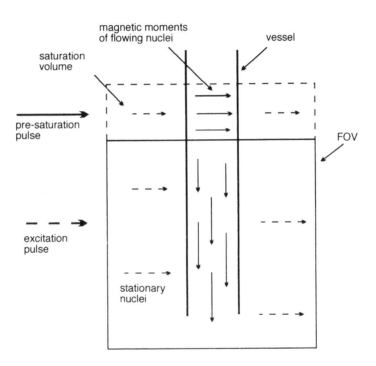

Fig. 6.9 Pre-saturation.

To be effective, pre-saturation pulses should be placed between the flow and the imaging stack so that signal from flowing nuclei entering the FOV is nullified. In sagittal and axial imaging, pre-saturation pulses are usually placed above and below the FOV so that arterial flow from above, and venous flow from below is saturated. Right and left pre-saturation pulses are sometimes useful in coronal imaging (especially in the chest), to saturate flow from the subclavian vessels.

Software available on most systems allows pre-saturation pulses to be brought into the FOV itself. This permits artefact producing areas (such as the aorta) to be pre-saturated so that phase mismapping can be reduced (Chapter 7).

Pre-saturation pulses are only useful if they are applied to tissue. If they are applied to air they are not effective. They increase the amount of RF that is delivered to the patient, which may increase heating effects (Chapter 10). The use of pre-saturation pulses may also decrease the number of slices available and should therefore be used appropriately.

Pre-saturation pulses are also only effective if the flowing nucleus receives the 90° pre-saturation pulse. Pulses are applied around each slice just before the excitation pulse. The TR, and the number of slices, therefore govern the interval between the delivery of each pre-saturation pulse. To optimise pre-saturation, use all the slices permitted for a given TR. As pre-saturation produces a signal void, it is usually used in T1 and proton density weighted images where fluid (blood and CSF), is dark anyway. Figure 6.10 shows axial T1 weighted gradient echo images of the abdomen with and without pre-saturation.

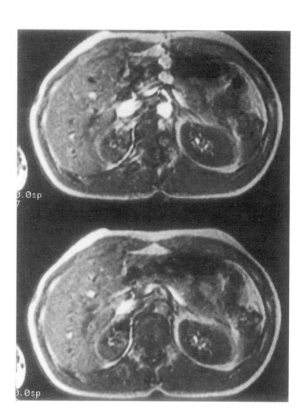

Fig. 6.10 Axial T1 weighted gradient echo images of the abdomen. The upper image demonstrates artefact from flowing nuclei within the aorta. The lower image uses pre-saturation volumes placed superior and inferior to the slice, to reduce the artefact.

Other uses of pre-saturation

Pre-saturation nullifies signal and can therefore be used to specifically eliminate certain signals. The main uses of this are:

(1) fat and water saturation,
(2) to reduce aliasing.

Fat and water saturation

Hydrogen exists in different chemical environments in the body which include fat and water. In fat, hydrogen is linked to carbon and in water it is linked to oxygen. The precessional frequency of fat is slightly different from that of water. As the main magnetic field strength increases, this frequency difference also increases. For example at 1.5 T, the precessional frequency between fat and water is approximately 220 Hz, so fat precesses at 220 Hz less than water. At 1.0 T this frequency difference is reduced to 147 Hz. In order to saturate either fat or water, the precessional difference between the two must be sufficiently large so that they can be isolated from each other. Fat or water saturation is therefore most effectively achieved on high field systems.

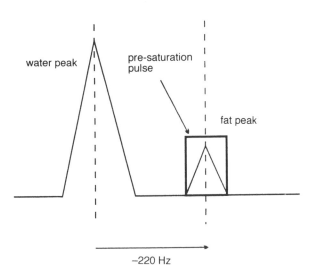

Fig. 6.11 Fat saturation.

To saturate fat signal, a 90° pre-saturation pulse must be applied at the precessional frequency of fat to the whole FOV (Fig. 6.11). The excitation RF pulse is then applied to the slices and the magnetic moments of the fat nuclei are flipped into saturation. If they are flipped to 180°, they do not have a component of transverse magnetisation and produce a signal void. The water nuclei however are excited, rephased and produce a signal. Figure 6.12 compares sagittal T1 weighted images of the lumbar spine, with and without fat pre-saturation.

To saturate water signal, the pre-saturation pulse must be applied at the precessional frequency of water to the whole FOV (Fig. 6.13). The RF excitation pulse is then applied to the slices, and the magnetic moments of nuclei in water are flipped into saturation. If they are flipped to 180°, they do not have a transverse component of magnetisation and produce a signal void. The fat nuclei however are excited, rephased and produce a signal. Figure 6.14 compares axial T1 weighted images of the liver, with and without water pre-saturation.

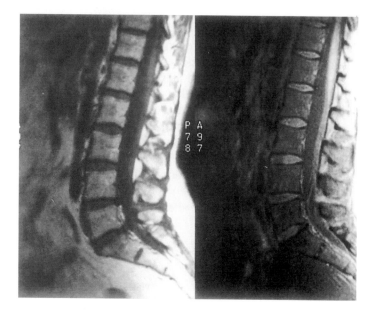

Fig. 6.12 Sagittal T1 weighted images of the lumbar spine without fat pre-saturation (left), and with fat pre-saturation (right).

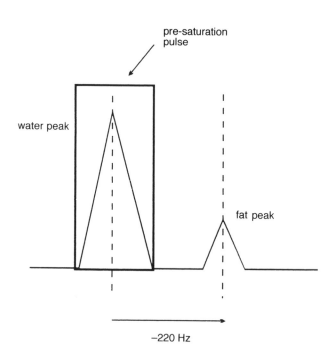

Fig. 6.13 Water saturation.

Uses of fat and water pre-saturation

Fat saturation has many uses, but distinguishing between the fatty and non-fatty components of tumour is probably the most important. Water saturation may be used to estimate the fat content of liver.

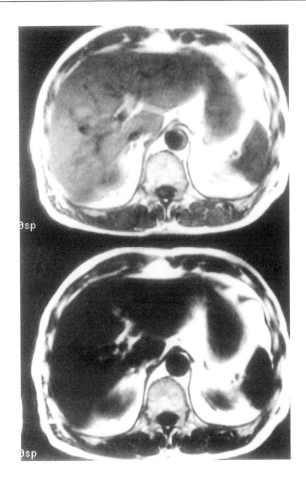

Fig. 6.14 Axial T1 weighted images of the abdomen without water pre-saturation (above), and with water pre-saturation (below). Note how the signal intensity is reduced in the liver on the lower image.

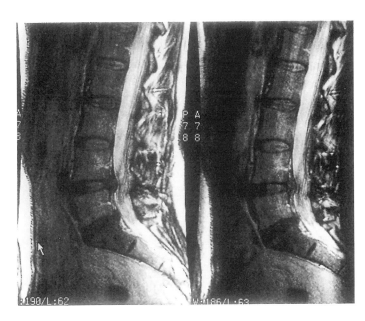

Fig. 6.15 Sagittal T2 weighted images of the lumbar spine using rectangular FOV. The high signal bands anterior (arrow), and posterior are phase wrap. Pre-saturation volumes placed over this artefact reduce its effect.

To be used effectively, there should be an even distribution of fat or water throughout the FOV. Pre-saturation RF is transmitted at the same frequency and evenly to the whole FOV, so that a particularly dense area of fat receives the same pre-saturation energy as an area with very little fat. Under these circumstances fat saturation is less effective. In addition, the gradients applied for spatial encoding vary the frequency across each slice. For this reason chemical pre-saturation often appears non-uniform across the slice or imaging volume. Therefore optimal saturation occurs at the centre of a slice or in the central portion of the imaging volume. Fat and water pre-saturation delivers extra RF into the patient and therefore reduces the number of slices available for a given TR.

The pre-saturation pulses are delivered to the FOV before the excitation of each slice. The interval between the pre-saturation pulses is called the SAT TR and is equal to the scan TR divided by the number of slices. If the SAT TR is longer than the T1 times of fat or water, the NMV's of fat or water may not be saturated as they have had time to recover before each pre-saturation pulse is delivered. To prevent this, always prescribe the maximum number of slices available for a given TR so that the SAT TR is reduced to a minimum.

Pre-saturation to prevent aliasing

Aliasing is produced when anatomy exists outside the FOV. It can be eliminated by using anti-aliasing methods as described in Chapter 7. However pre-saturation can help to reduce the signal from tissue outside the FOV, so the effect of aliasing is less pronounced (Fig. 6.15).

Even echo rephasing

If two or more echoes are produced in a spin echo pulse sequence, intra-voxel dephasing may be reduced by acquiring the second and succeeding even echoes at a multiple of the first TE, for example, two echoes, first TE 40 ms and second TE 80 ms. This works on the principle that flowing nuclei that are out of phase at the first echo, are in phase at the second echo as long as the nuclei are given exactly the same amount of time to rephase as they were given to dephase. In other words, if at the first TE of 40 ms they are out of phase, 40 ms later (at 80 ms) they will be in phase again. This is called *even echo rephasing* and can be used to reduce artefact in a T2 weighted image.

- Gradient moment rephasing:
    uses additional gradients to correct altered phase values,
    reduces artefact from intra-voxel dephasing,
    gives flowing nuclei a bright signal,
    is mainly used in T2 or T2* weighted images,
    is most effective on slow, laminar flow within the slice.

- Pre-saturation:

  uses additional RF pulses to nullify signal from flowing nuclei,
  reduces artefact due to time of flight and entry slice phenomenon,
  gives flowing nuclei a signal void,
  is mainly used in T1 weighted images,
  is effective on fast and slow flow,
  increases the RF deposition to the patient,
  can be used to nullify signal from fat or water and to reduce aliasing.

Now that flow phenomena have been discussed it is appropriate to proceed to explore other artefacts that are commonly seen on MR images. These are described in the next chapter.

Questions

1. What time of flight RF pulsing circumstances create a signal void in spin echo sequences?

2. Why are vessels usually bright on gradient echo sequences?

3. Will arterial flow be co/counter current on an axial brain acquisition scanning from foot to head?

4. In an axial acquisition of the abdomen when slices are acquired from the feet to the head with no pre-saturation of gradient moment nulling on the most inferior slice:
   (a) the aorta will be bright and the inferior vena cava dark
   (b) the aorta will be dark and the inferior vena cava bright
   (c) the aorta and the inferior vena cava will be bright.

5. What is pre-saturation? Where would you place pre-saturation volumes on a small FOV coronal left shoulder?

6. When would you use gradient moment nulling?

Chapter 7 Artefacts and Their Compensation

Introduction

All MRI images have artefacts to some degree. It is therefore very important that the causes of these artefacts are understood and compensated for if possible. Some artefacts are irreversible, and may only be reduced rather than eliminated. Others can be avoided altogether. This chapter discusses the causes and remedy of the most common artefacts encountered in MRI.

Phase mismapping

Phase mismapping is produced by anatomy moving along a gradient during the pulse sequence. It can happen along any gradient. Let us assume for the purposes of this explanation that anatomy is moving across the phase encoding gradient.

In Fig. 7.1 the chest wall is located at position A during one phase encoding (expiration), but may have moved to position B during the next phase encoding (inspiration). The chest wall is given a phase value associated with position A during the first phase encoding, (12 o'clock). Another phase value (3 o'clock), associated with position B along the gradient, is given at the next phase encoding step. In this way moving anatomy is mismapped into the FOV.

An artefact known as *ghosting* is produced, and originates from any structure that moves during the acquisition of data, for example, chest wall during respiration, pulsatile movement of vessels, swallowing, eye movement. Phase mismapping always occurs along the phase encoding axis. This is due to the inherent time delay between phase encoding and readout and motion between each phase encode (Fig. 7.2). No mismapping occurs along the frequency axis as frequency encoding is performed as the signal is read and the amplitude of the frequency encode

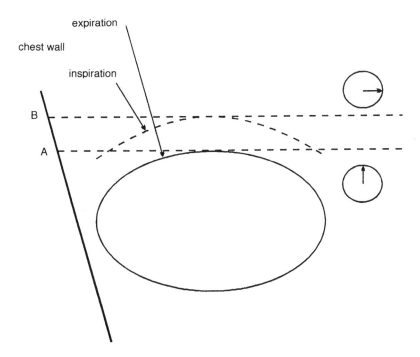

Fig. 7.1   How ghosting occurs.

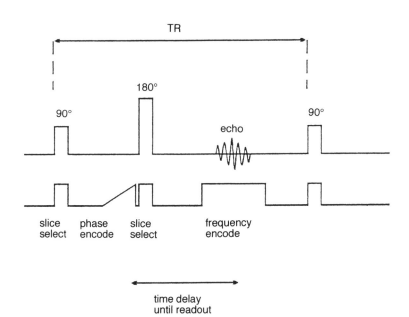

Fig. 7.2   Time delay between phase encoding and readout.

remains constant. When looking at an image, the direction of phase encoding can always be determined by the direction of the phase mismapping or ghosting artefact. Figure 7.3 shows an axial image of the abdomen with the ghosting artefact.

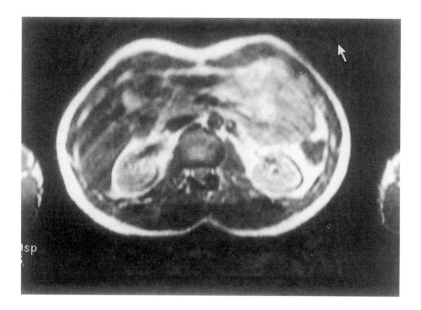

Fig. 7.3   Axial image of the abdomen. The arrow shows the ghosting artefact. What weighting is this image, and do you think ghosting will be worse on a T1 or a T2 weighted image?

The remedy

There are several ways of reducing phase mismapping. Total elimination, is however impossible unless of course you are imaging a cadaver! The remedies of mismapping are associated with their individual causes.

Remedy 1.   As ghosting only occurs along the phase axis, the direction of phase encoding can be changed, so that the artefact does not interfere with the area of interest.

For example in a sagittal lumbar spine, frequency encoding is usually performed by the Z gradient (head to foot) as this is the longest axis of the patient in the sagittal plane. Phase is therefore anterior posterior and performed by the Y gradient. Pulsatile motion of the aorta along the phase axis produces ghosting over the spinal cord. Swapping phase and frequency so that frequency encoding is performed by the Y gradient (anterior posterior), and the Z gradient performs phase encoding, places the artefact head to foot so that it does not obscure the spinal cord. This can be seen in Fig. 7.4.

This remedy is also useful in sagittal imaging of the knee to remove artefact originating from the popliteal artery, and in axial imaging of the chest where anterior mediastinal structures are obscured by the aorta.

Which way do you think phase and frequency should be located in these examples?

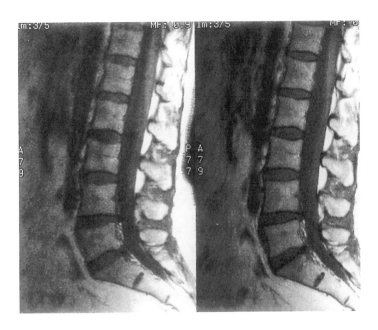

Fig. 7.4 Sagittal T1 weighted images of the lumbar spine swapping the phase direction. The image on the left has phase anterior posterior, as compared with the image on the right that has phase superior to inferior. Note that phase artefact obscures detail in the spinal cord on the first image, whereas swapping the phase axis to superior inferior on the second image, displaces the artefact away from the cord.

Remedy 2. A process known as pre-saturation was discussed in Chapter 6. Pre-saturation nulls signal from specified areas. Placing pre-saturation volumes over the area producing artefact nullifies signal and reduces the artefact.

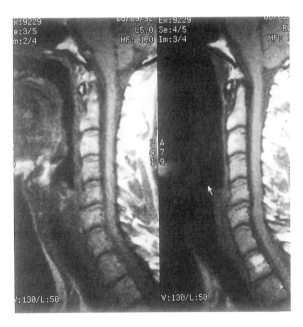

Fig. 7.5 Sagittal T1 weighted images of the cervical spine. The image on the left demonstrates how swallowing can degrade image quality. The image on the right has a saturation volume placed over the throat (arrow), and detail in the cord is demonstrated more clearly.

For example, in sagittal imaging of the cervical spine, swallowing produces ghosting along the phase axis (anterior posterior) and obscures the spinal cord. Bringing a pre-saturation pulse into the FOV and placing it over the throat reduces the artefact (Fig. 7.5).

In addition, pre-saturation reduces artefact from flowing nuclei in blood vessels. Pre-saturation produces low signal from these nuclei and is most effective when placed between the origin of the flow and the FOV.

Remedy 3. When imaging the chest and abdomen, respiratory motion along the phase axis produces phase mismapping. Most sequences are not short enough to permit the patient to hold their breath during data acquisition, and so this motion must be compensated for in some way.

Most systems have a method known as *respiratory compensation* that greatly reduces ghosting from respiration. This entails placing a set of bellows around the patient's chest when imaging the chest or abdomen. These bellows are corrugated in their middle portion and expand and contract as the patient breathes. This expansion and contraction causes air to move back and forth through the bellows. The bellows are connected by hollow rubber tubing to a transducer located on the system (Fig. 7.6). A transducer is a device that converts the mechanical motion of air flowing back and forth along the bellows to an electrical signal. The system therefore analyses this signal, the amplitude of which corresponds to the maximum and minimum motion of the chest wall during respiration.

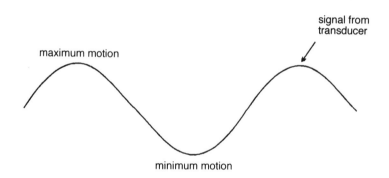

Fig. 7.6 The respiratory signal.

Respiratory compensation and K space filling

As described in Chapter 3, the central lines of K space are filled after shallow phase encoding gradient slopes (which result in good SNR), whereas the outer lines are filled after steep phase encoding gradient slopes that result in high spatial resolution. Anatomy that moves along a steep phase encoding slope, produces maximum ghosting as there is a large phase shift between A and B. Anatomy that moves along a shallow phase encoding gradient slope however, produces less ghosting as there is a smaller phase shift between A and B (Fig. 7.7). Shallow phase slopes also fill the centre of K space which provides the signal in the image.

The system is able to read the electrical signal from the transducer and perform the shallow phase encoding gradient slopes when the chest or

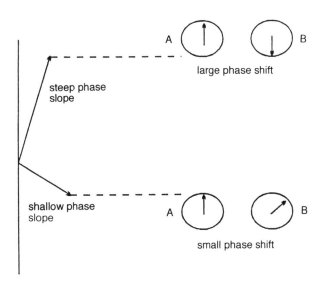

Fig. 7.7 Ghosting increases with the slope of the phase encoding gradient.

abdominal wall movement is at a minimum, so that most of the data which provides image signal and contrast is acquired when chest wall motion is low. It reserves the steep phase encoding slopes for when the chest wall movement is at a maximum (Fig. 7.8). In this way, the ghosting artefact from respiratory motion is reduced.

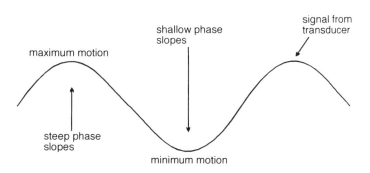

Fig. 7.8 Respiratory compensation.

Some systems use a method known as respiratory gating that times the excitation RF with a certain phase of respiration. Each slice of the acquisition is therefore obtained at the same phase of respiration. However, this method has several drawbacks. First, the TR and therefore the contrast is determined by the rapidity of respiration and secondly since respiratory rates are generally longer than the TR, the scan time is lengthened and image contrast may change. As a result this method of gated respiration is rarely used.

Respiratory compensation (or the respiratory ordered phase encoding method as it is sometimes known), does not affect the scan time or the image contrast (Fig. 7.9). The only penalty of this method is that the number of slices available for a given TR may be slightly reduced.

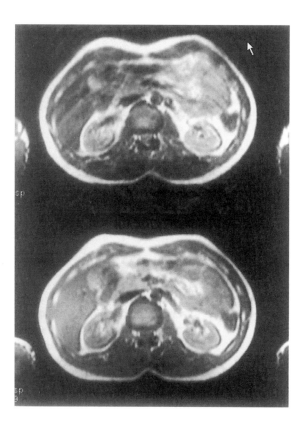

Fig. 7.9 Axial T1 weighted images of the abdomen without respiratory compensation (above), and using respiratory compensation (below). The ghosting (arrow), has been reduced on the lower image.

Remedy 4.   Gating is a very general term used to describe a technique of reducing phase mismapping from the periodic motion caused by respiration, cardiac, and pulsatile flow motion. Just as respiratory gating monitors respiration, cardiac gating monitors cardiac motion by co-ordinating the excitation pulse with the R wave of systole. This is achieved by using an electrical signal generated by the cardiac motion to trigger each excitation pulse. There are two forms of gating.

(1) *Electrocardiogram (ECG, EKG) gating* uses electrodes and lead wires that are attached to the patient's chest to produce an ECG. This is used to determine the timing of the application of each excitation pulse. Each slice is acquired at the same phase of the cardiac cycle and therefore phase mismapping from cardiac motion is reduced. ECG gating should be used when imaging the chest, heart and great vessels (Fig. 7.10).

(2) *Peripheral gating* uses a light sensor attached to the patient's finger to detect the pulsation of blood through the capillaries. The pulsation is used to trigger the excitation pulses so that each slice is acquired at the same phase of the cardiac cycle. Peripheral gating is not as accurate as ECG gating, so is not very useful when imaging the heart itself. However, it is effective at reducing phase mismapping when imaging small vessels or the spinal cord, where CSF flow may degrade the image. ECG and peripheral gating are discussed in more detail in Chapter 8.

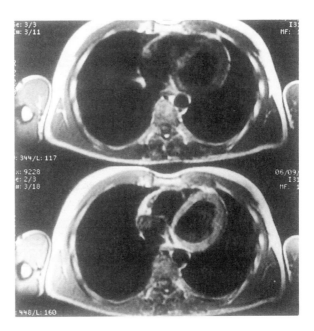

Fig. 7.10 Axial images of the chest without ECG gating (above), and with ECG gating (below). The anatomical detail of the heart is demonstrated clearly on the gated image.

Remedy 5. Gradient moment nulling (discussed in Chapter 6) reduces ghosting caused by flowing nuclei moving along gradients. It produces a bright signal from these flowing nuclei and also reduces ghosting significantly. It is most effective in slow, regular flow within the imaging plane.

Aliasing or wrap around

Aliasing is an artefact produced when anatomy that exists outside the FOV is mapped inside the FOV. Anatomy outside the selected FOV, still produces a signal if it is in close proximity to the receiver coil. Data from this signal must be encoded, i.e. it must be allocated a pixel position. If the data is under sampled, the signal is mismapped into pixels within the FOV rather than outside. This is called *aliasing* or *wrap around*, as the anatomy outside the FOV is folded into the selected FOV. Aliasing can occur along both the frequency and phase axis.

Frequency wrap

Aliasing along the frequency encoding axis is known as frequency wrap. This is caused by under sampling the frequencies that are present in the echo. These frequencies originate from any signal, regardless of whether the anatomy producing it is inside or outside the selected FOV. Ideally, only the frequencies originating from inside the FOV are allocated a pixel position. This only occurs if the frequencies are sampled often enough. According to the Nyquist theorem (Chapter 3), frequencies must be sampled at least twice per cycle in order to map them correctly. If the Nyquist theorem is not obeyed, the frequencies are under sampled and signal from anatomy outside the FOV in the frequency encoding direction is mapped into the FOV (Fig. 7.11). Wrap around results along the frequency encoding axis.

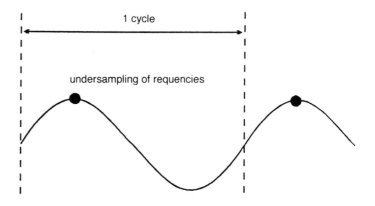

Fig. 7.11 Under sampling of frequencies.

Phase wrap

Aliasing along the phase axis of the image is known as phase wrap. This is caused by under sampling along the phase axis. After FFT every phase value from 0–360° (or 12 o'clock through to the following 12 o'clock) must be mapped into the FOV in the phase encoding direction (Fig. 7.12). This phase curve is repeated on both sides of the FOV along the phase axis. Any signal is allocated a phase value according to its position along this curve. As the curve is repeated, signal originating outside the FOV in the phase direction is allocated a phase value that has already been given to signal originating from inside the FOV. There is, therefore, a duplication of phase values. This duplication causes phase wrap along the phase axis.

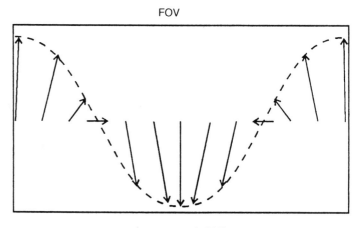

Fig. 7.12 The phase curve.

For example, signal coming from X has the same phase value as signal coming from Y, as they both share the same position along the phase curve. Anatomy from X is mapped over anatomy at Y (Figs 7.13 and 7.14).

Aliasing along both the frequency and phase axis can totally degrade an image and should be compensated for. Enlarging the FOV so that all the

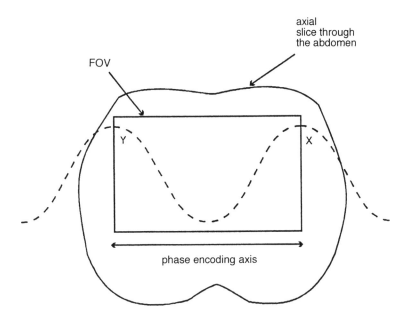

Fig. 7.13 X and Y have the same value of phase.

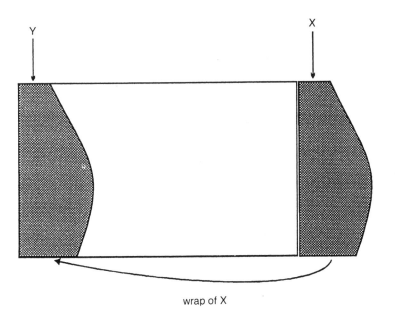

wrap of X

Fig. 7.14 Phase wrap.

anatomy producing signal is incorporated within the FOV achieves this but also results in a loss of spatial resolution. There are however, two anti aliasing methods available that compensate for wrap.

Anti-aliasing along the frequency axis

This is often termed *no frequency wrap*. No frequency wrap uses digital RF pulses to cut off signal frequencies at the edges of the FOV along the frequency encoding axis. Signal originating from outside the FOV along the frequency axis is no longer mismapped as it is filtered out of the echo (Fig. 7.15). Most systems automatically apply no frequency wrap.

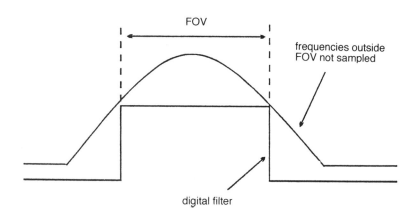

Fig. 7.15 Anti-aliasing along the frequency axis.

Anti-aliasing along the phase axis

This is often termed *no phase wrap*. No phase wrap over samples along the phase encoding axis by increasing the number of phase encodings performed. This is achieved by enlarging the FOV in the phase direction so that the phase curve extends over a wider area of anatomy. There is now no duplication of phase values as signal outside the FOV has a different phase value to that inside – anatomy is no longer mismapped and aliasing does not occur (Figs 7.16 and 7.17). However, as enlarging the FOV results in a loss of spatial resolution, the number of phase encodings is increased to compensate for this. Increasing the number of phase encodings in turn, increases the scan time and so some systems automatically reduce the NEX to compensate for this. There is however no noticeable reduction in SNR, as the increased number of phase encodings results in more data collection, which tends to offset the reduction in NEX. The extended portion of the FOV is usually discarded during reconstruction so that only the selected FOV is displayed (Fig. 7.16).

Although the SNR is not noticeably reduced, image quality may suffer slightly with no phase wrap. As a decrease in NEX reduces the number of signal averages, motion artefacts may be more apparent.

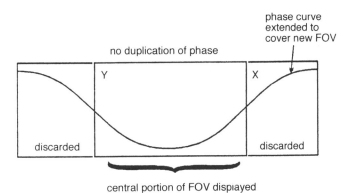

phase curve
extended to
cover new FOV

no duplication of phase

Y

X

discarded

discarded

Fig. 7.16 Anti-aliasing along
the phase axis.

central portion of FOV displayed

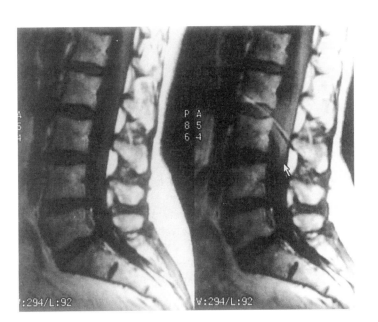

Fig. 7.17 Sagittal T1
weighted images of the
lumbar spine. The artefact
(arrow) is phase wrap. The
image on the left was acquired
using anti-aliasing measures.

No phase wrap and K space

Analysing how no phase wrap alters K space filling, provides a rather
'back to front' approach to understanding anti-aliasing, but the principles
are exactly the same. As discussed in Chapter 3, the incremental step
between each phase encoding gradient slope is inversely proportional to
the FOV in the phase direction. No phase wrap uses the more steep
phase encoding gradients to maintain spatial resolution and to over
sample along the phase axis. In order to do this and occupy the same
dimensions of K space, the incremental step between each phase
encoding gradient slope must be reduced. Reducing this increment
increases the FOV in the phase direction due to the inverse proportionality between the two factors (Fig. 7.18).

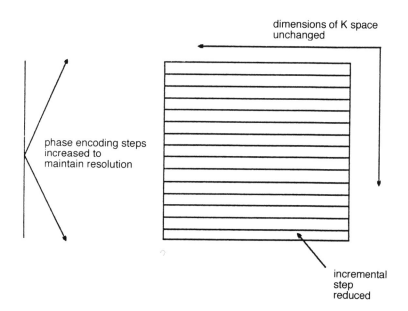

dimensions of K space
unchanged

phase encoding steps
increased to
maintain resolution

incremental
step
reduced

Fig. 7.18 Anti-aliasing
(phase) and K space filling.

Chemical shift artefact

Chemical shift artefact is caused by the different chemical environments of fat and water. Although fat and water are both made up of hydrogen protons, fat consists of hydrogen linked to carbon, whereas water hydrogen is linked to oxygen. As a result, fat precesses at a lower frequency than water. This difference in precessional frequency is proportional to the main magnetic field strength B_0, for example, at 1.5 T the difference in precessional frequency is 220 Hz. That is, fat precesses 220 Hz less than water. At 1.0 T this difference is 147 Hz and at lower field strengths (0.5 T or less), it is usually insignificant. However at higher field strengths, it can lead to an artefact known as *chemical shift*. The amount of chemical shift is often expressed in arbitrary units known as parts per million (ppm) of the main magnetic field strength. It's value is always independent of the main field strength and equals 3.5 ppm. From this, the chemical shift between fat and water can be calculated at different field strengths.

The receive bandwidth determines the range of frequencies that must be mapped across the FOV. The FOV is divided into pixels, the number of which is determined by the matrix size. If 256 frequency samples are selected, the receive bandwidth must be mapped across 256 pixels in the FOV. The receive bandwidth and the number of frequency samples determine the bandwidth of each pixel or frequency column (Fig. 7.19).

For example, if the receive bandwidth is ± 16 KHz, 32 000 Hz are mapped across the FOV. If 256 frequency samples are collected, the FOV is divided into 256 frequency columns or pixels. Each column therefore has an individual frequency range of 125 Hz per pixel (32 000/256 Hz).

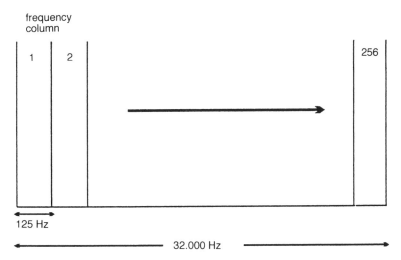

Fig. 7.19 Frequency per pixel.

At a field strength of 1.5 T, the precessional frequency difference between fat and water is 220 Hz and therefore using the above example, fat and water protons existing adjacent to one other in the patient are mapped 1.76 pixels apart (220/125) (Fig. 7.20). This pixel shift of fat relative to water is called chemical shift artefact. The actual dimensions of this artefact depend on the size of the FOV as this determines the size of each pixel.

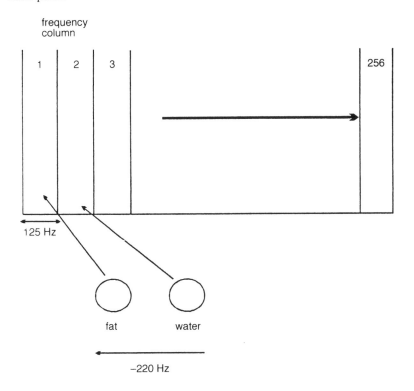

Fig. 7.20 Chemical shift at 1.5 T.

For example, a FOV of 24 cm and 256 frequency columns results in pixels 0.93 mm in size. A pixel shift of 1.76 results in an actual chemical shift between fat and water of 1.63 mm (0.93 × 1.76 mm). As the FOV is enlarged this dimension increases.

Chemical shift artefact causes a dark edge at the interface between fat and water. It occurs along the frequency encoding axis only.

The remedy

Chemical shift can be limited by scanning at lower field strengths and by keeping the FOV to a minimum. At high field strengths, the size of the receive bandwidth is one way of limiting chemical shift. As the receive bandwidth is reduced, a smaller frequency range must now be mapped across the same number of frequency columns, for example, 256. The individual frequency range of each pixel therefore decreases, and so the 220 Hz difference in precessional frequency between fat and water is translated into a larger pixel shift (Fig. 7.21).

For example, if the receive bandwidth is reduced to ±8 kHz, only 16 000 Hz is now mapped across 256 frequency columns. Each pixel has

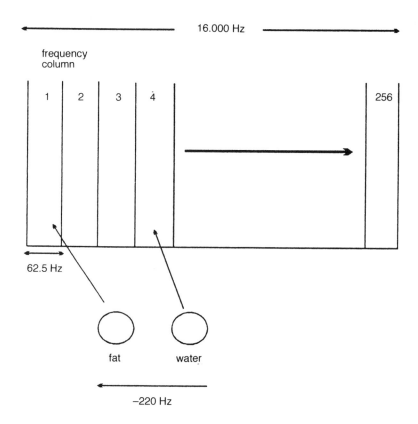

Fig. 7.21 Chemical shift at reduced bandwidth.

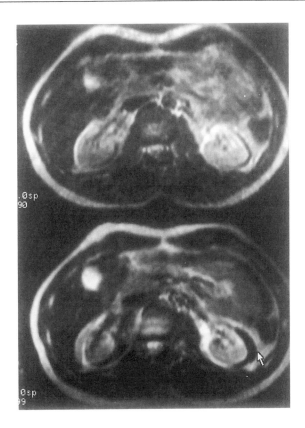

Fig. 7.22 Axial T2 weighted images of the abdomen using a receive bandwidth of 32 000 Hz (above), and 8 000 Hz (below). The arrow demonstrates chemical shift artefact at the border of the left kidney.

a range of only 62.5 Hz (16 000/256 Hz). The 220 Hz precessional frequency difference between the two adjacent fat and water protons, is now translated into a pixel shift of 3.52 pixels (220/62.5) (Fig. 7.22).

To reduce chemical shift artefact always use the widest receive bandwidth in keeping with good SNR and the smallest FOV possible. If the bandwidth is reduced to increase the SNR, use chemical saturation to saturate out the signal from either fat or water (Chapter 6). These measures are really only necessary at higher field strengths. At 0.5 T or less, chemical shift artefact is insignificant and usually does not need to be compensated for.

Chemical misregistration

Chemical misregistration is an artefact also produced as a result of the precessional frequency difference between fat and water. However, in this case, the artefact is caused because fat and water are in phase at certain times and out of phase at others, due to the difference in their precessional frequency. As they travel at different speeds around their precessional paths, they are at various positions on the path but periodically they are at the same position and therefore in phase.

LEARNING POINT

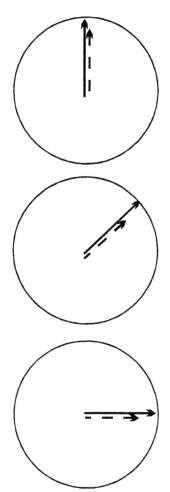

This is analogous to the hour and minute hand of a clock. Both hands travel at different speeds around the clock; the hour hand moves through 360° in 12 h, whereas the minute hand moves the same distance in 1 h. However at certain times of the day, the hands are superimposed or in phase, i.e. at 12 noon, 1.05 AM, 2.10 AM, 3.15 AM etc. (Fig. 7.23).

When fat and water are in phase their signals add constructively, and when they are out of phase their signals cancel each other out (Fig. 7.24). This cancellation effect is known as *chemical misregistration* artefact, which causes a ring of dark signal around certain organs where fat and water interfaces occur within the same voxel, for example, the kidneys (Fig. 7.25). Chemical misregistration mainly occurs in the phase direction, as it is produced due to a phase difference between fat and water. It is most degrading to the image in gradient echo pulse sequences, where gradient reversal is very ineffective. In spin echo sequences, the 180° rephasing pulse compensates for the phase difference between fat and water, and so chemical misregistration artefact is reduced.

The remedy

Use a spin echo sequence to reduce the artefact. In gradient echo pulse sequences select a TE that corresponds to the periodicity of fat and water. In other words, select a TE that generates an echo when fat and water are in phase, so that their signals add constructively. The periodicity of fat and water depends on the field strength. At 1.5 T for example, selecting a TE that is a multiple of 4.2 ms reduces chemical misregistration artefact, whereas at 0.5 T the periodicity of fat and water is 7 ms.

For example, at a TE of 8.4 ms there is little artefact, but at a TE of 10.4 ms chemical misregistration occurs.

Fig. 7.23 The hands of a clock are in phase at certain times of the day and out of phase at others.

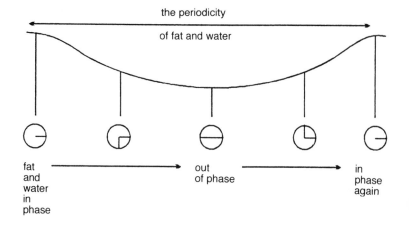

the periodicity of fat and water

fat and water in phase   out of phase   in phase again

Fig. 7.24 The periodicity of fat and water.

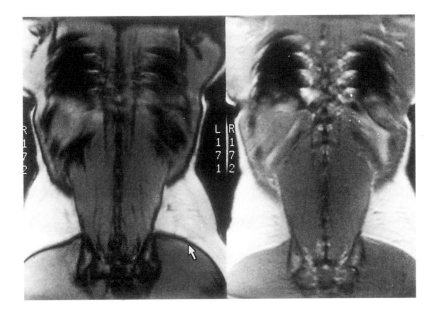

Fig. 7.25 Coronal T1 weighted gradient echo images of the posterior abdomen acquired on a 1.5 T system. The image on the left was acquired with a TE of 2.8 ms, whereas the image on the right has a TE of 4.2 ms. The arrow shows chemical misregistration artefact.

Truncation artefact

This artefact results from under sampling of data so that interfaces of high and low signal are incorrectly represented on the image. A common site for this artefact is in T1 sagittal imaging of the cervical spine, where there

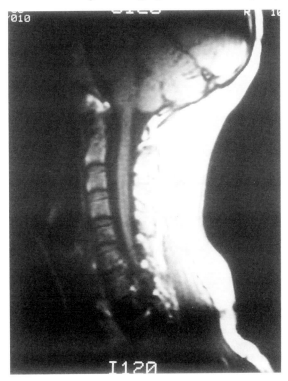

Fig. 7.26 Sagittal T1 weighted image of the cervical spine using an image matrix of 256 × 128. The dark line in the cord is truncation (Gibbs) artefact.

is low signal from the CSF and high signal from the spinal cord. This is specifically called Gibbs artefact. Truncation artefact occurs in the phase direction only and produces a low intensity band running through a high intensity area (Fig. 7.26).

The remedy

The under sampling of data must be avoided. To do so, increase the number of phase encoding steps.

For example, use 256 × 256 matrix instead of 256 × 128.

Magnetic susceptibility artefact

Magnetic susceptibility is the ability of a substance to become magnetised. Some tissues magnetise to different degrees than others, which results in a difference in precessional frequency and phase. This causes dephasing at

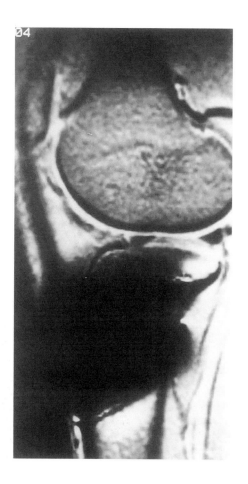

Fig. 7.27 Sagittal gradient echo sequence of the knee. Magnetic susceptibility artefact from the screws degrades the image.

the interface of these tissues and a signal loss. In practice, the main causes of this artefact are metal and the iron content of haemorrhage, as these magnetise to a much greater degree than the surrounding tissue. Ferromagnetic objects have a very high magnetic susceptibility and cause distortion of the image. Magnetic susceptibility artefact is more prominent in gradient echo sequences as the gradient reversal cannot compensate for the phase difference at the interface (Fig. 7.27).

The remedy

Always ensure that the patient has removed all metal items where possible before the scan. Always check whether the patient has aneurysm clips or metal implants. Most implants can be scanned, but may cause local heating effects (see Chapter 10). When imaging in the vicinity of a metal implant the artefact may obscure the anatomy under examination. The use of spin echo sequences reduces the artefact. Magnetic susceptibility artefact can be used to aid diagnosis in the case of haemorrhage. The artefact causes a signal void if an area of abnormality contains old blood.

Zipper artefact

Zipper artefact appears as a dense line on the image at a specific point. This is caused by extraneous RF entering the room at a certain frequency, and interfering with the inherently weak signal coming from the patient. It is caused by a leak in the RF shielding of the room (Fig. 7.28).

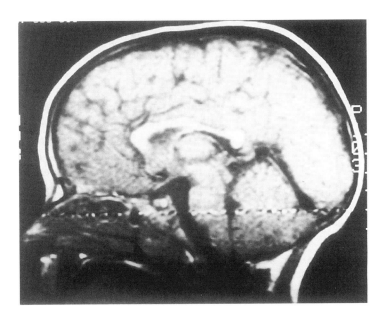

Fig. 7.28 Sagittal T1 weighted image of the brain. The line across the image represents interference at a certain frequency.

The remedy

Call the engineer to locate the leak and repair it.

Shading artefact

Shading is an artefact which produces a loss of signal intensity in one part of the image. Its main cause is the uneven excitation of nuclei within the patient due to RF pulses applied at flip angles other than 90° and 180°. Shading is also caused by abnormal loading on the coil or by coupling of the coil at one point. This may occur with a large patient, who touches one side of the body coil and couples it at that point.

Shading can also be caused by inhomogeneities in the main magnetic field which can be improved by shimming (see Chapter 9).

The remedy

Always ensure that the coil is loaded correctly, i.e. that the correct size of coil is used for the anatomy under examination, and that the patient is not touching the coil at any point. The use of foam pads or water bags between the coil and the patient will usually suffice. In addition, also ensure that appropriate pre-scan parameters have been obtained before the scan (see Chapter 3), as these determine the correct excitation frequency and amplitude of the applied RF pulses.

Motion of the patient

Any motion of the patient causes artefact. Motion is usually either involuntary (twitching, pulsation, bowel motion), or voluntary (swallowing nervousness), and causes image degradation.

The remedy

Involuntary motion can often be compensated for. Bowel motion can be reduced by giving the patient an anti-spasmodic agent prior to the scan when imaging the abdomen or pelvis. Pulsation can be reduced by the use of pre-saturation, gating or gradient moment nulling techniques. Increasing the NEX may also help, as this increases the number of times the signal is averaged (Fig. 7.29). Motion artefact is averaged out of the image as it is more random in nature than the signal itself. Voluntary motion can be reduced by making the patient as comfortable as possible, and immobilising them with pads and straps. A nervous patient always benefits from thoughtful explanation of the procedure, and a constant reminder over the system intercom to keep still. A relative or friend in the room can also help in some circumstances. In extreme cases, sedation of the patient may be required.

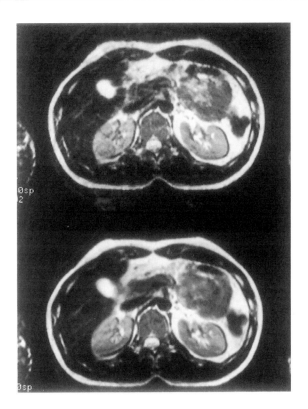

Fig. 7.29 Axial T2 weighted images of the abdomen using 1 NEX (above) and 4 NEX (below). The lower image shows less ghosting artefact.

Cross excitation and cross talk

An RF excitation pulse is not exactly square. The width of the pulse should be half its amplitude, but this normally varies by up to 10%. As a result, nuclei in slices adjacent to the RF excitation pulse may become excited by it. Adjacent slices receive energy from the RF excitation pulse of their neighbours (Fig. 7.30).

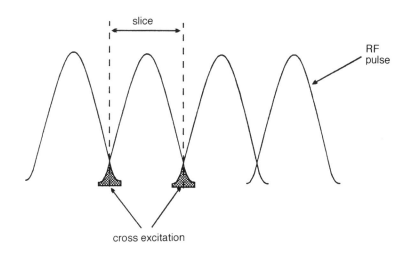

Fig. 7.30 Cross excitation.

This energy pushes the NMV of the nuclei towards the transverse plane, so that they may become saturated when they themselves are excited. This effect is called *cross excitation* and affects image contrast. The same effect is produced by energy dissipation to adjacent slices, as nuclei within the selected slice relax to B_0. These nuclei lose their energy due to spin lattice relaxation and may dissipate this energy to nuclei in neighbouring slices. This is specifically called *cross talk* and should not be confused with cross excitation.

The remedy

Cross talk can never be eliminated as it is caused by the natural dissipation of energy by the nuclei. Cross excitation can be reduced by ensuring that there is at least a 30% gap between the slices. This is 30% of the slice thickness itself, and reduces the likelihood of RF exciting adjacent slices. For example, if the slice thickness selected is 5 mm use a skip or gap of 2 mm (40% of 5 mm), rather than a 1 mm gap (20% of 5 mm). In addition, most systems excite alternate slices during the acquisition so that there is some time for cross excitation in adjacent slices to decay before it is their turn to be excited.

For example; excitation order of slices is 1, 3, 5, 7, 2, 4, 6, 8. Slices 1 to 7 have time to decay their cross excitation, while slices 2 to 8 are being excited (approximately half the TR).

A process known as *interleaving* extends this time even further. When interleaving slices, alternate slices are excited and divided into two acquisitions. In this way, cross excitation created in adjacent slices has the time of a whole acquisition to decay before it is its turn to be excited.

For example; excitation order of slices is 1, 3, 5, 7 in the first acquisition and 2, 4, 6, 8 in the second. Slices 1 to 7 have the time of a whole acquisition (several minutes) to decay, while slices 2 to 8 are being excited. When using interleaving, no gap is required between the slices.

Some systems use software to 'square off' the RF pulses so that the adjacent nuclei are less likely to become excited. This reduces cross excitation but often results in some loss of signal, as a proportion of the RF pulse is lost in the squaring off process. It is still wise to use a small gap of 10%, when employing this software.

There are some other artefacts caused by major equipment malfunction. The loss of a gradient for example causes distortion of the image, and eddy currents induced in the gradient coils can cause phase artefacts as they create additional unwanted phase shifts. On the whole however, artefacts produced in MR can be compensated for to some extent, and this is summarised in Table 7.1.

Table 7.1 Artefacts and their remedies.

Artefacts	Axis	Remedy	Penalty
Truncation	phase	increase phase encodings	increase scan time
Phase mismapping	phase	respiratory compensation	may lose a slice
		swap phase and frequency	may need no phase wrap
		gating	variable TR variable image contrast increased scan time
		pre-saturation	may lose a slice
		gradient moment rephasing	increases minimum TE
Chemical shift	frequency	increase bandwidth	decrease minimum TE available decrease SNR
		reduce FOV	reduces SNR decreases resolution
		use chemical saturation	reduces SNR may lose slices
Chemical misregistration	phase	select TE at periodicity of fat and water	may lose a slice if TE is increased significantly
Aliasing	frequency and phase	no frequency wrap	none
		no phase wrap	may reduce SNR may increase scan time with some vendors increases motion artefact due to reduced NEX
		enlarge the FOV	reduces resolution
Zipper	frequency	call engineer	irate engineer!
Magnetic susceptibility	frequency and phase	use spin echo	not flow sensitive blood product may be missed
		remove metal where possible	none
Shading	frequency and phase	check shim load coil correctly prescan correctly	none

continued

Table 7.1 *continued*

Artefacts	Axis	Remedy	Penalty
Motion	phase	use anti-spasmodics	costly, invasive
		immobilise patient	none
		counselling of patient	none
		all remedies for mismapping	see previous
		sedation	possible side effects invasive, costly requires monitoring
Cross talk	slice select	none	none
Cross excitation	slice select	interleaving	doubles the scan time
		squaring off RF pulses	reduces SNR

Questions

1. What is truncation artefact and how would you try and rectify it?

2. You are examining a knee with a prosthesis *in situ*. What artefact would you expect to see, and how would you try to achieve the optimum image quality?

3. What is the difference between chemical shift and chemical misregistration?

4. Under what conditions would you get phase wrap?

5. How is K space filling altered in:
   (a) anti-aliasing/no phase wrap?
   (b) respiratory compensation?

6. What is the difference between cross talk and cross excitation? Which can be reduced and how?

7. List the different motion compensation options.

Chapter 8   Vascular and Cardiac Imaging

Introduction

There are several methods which can be used to evaluate both the neurovascular and cardiovascular systems with the use of MRI. A series of magnetic resonance vascular imaging techniques are available to evaluate non-invasively both the morphology and haemodynamics of the vascular system. Such techniques include conventional MRI (acquired with imaging options to enable vascular visualisation) and Magnetic Resonance Angiography – MRA – (acquired to visualise moving blood). Prior to MRA, the patient would be required to undergo both conventional angiographic and/or cardiac catheterization procedures to study vascular anatomy, as well as Doppler ultrasound to study flow velocity and direction. MRI enables direct imaging correlation between haemodynamic flow velocity and morphologic display, with little or no discomfort to the patient or to the radiographer. The current techniques used are now discussed.

Conventional vascular imaging techniques

These techniques involve using options such as gradient moment rephasing and pre-saturation. As previously discussed in Chapter 6, they are used to reduce motion artefact from flowing nuclei. However, as they give nuclei flowing in blood either signal void or signal enhancement, they also produce contrast between vessels and the surrounding tissue. These techniques can therefore be very useful to demonstrate occlusion of a vessel, if the more recent angiographic procedures are not available. Pre-saturation and gradient moment rephasing are now described in the context of vascular imaging.

Black blood imaging

To give an anatomic structure contrast relative to other tissues within the body, the structure must appear either darker or brighter than the

183

surrounding tissues. Several techniques can be employed to produce images where vessels appear dark. These include spin echo acquisitions and the application of pre-saturation pulses. In spin echo sequences, rapidly flowing blood appears dark enabling visualisation of the vessel relative to surrounding tissues. Nuclei that receive both the 90° and 180° pulses will produce an MR signal. However, flowing nuclei that receive either the 90° pulse or the 180° pulse (but not both) produce no signal. When spin echo acquisitions produce images where blood is dark they can be referred to as *black blood images* (Fig. 8.1). This technique can be further improved by the application of pre-saturation pulses (see Chapter 6). Short TR/TE spin echo imaging with the use of pre-saturation pulses, enables visualisation of the vascular system in that flowing vessels appear black. Saturation eliminates phase ghosting and provides intra-luminal signal void for excellent distinction between patent and obstructed vessels.

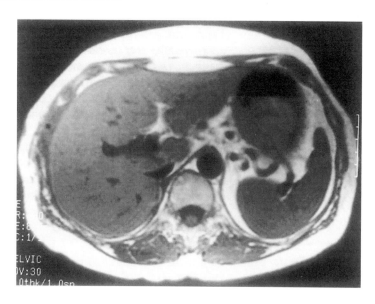

Fig. 8.1 This axial image of the liver was acquired with a spin echo. Note the low signal intensity arising from the abdominal vessels.

Pre-saturation can be used to evaluate vascular patency throughout the head and body. However since pre-saturation uses additional RF pulses, the specific absorption rate (SAR, discussed in Chapter 10) is increased, and the slice number available per TR may be reduced as a result. Additional pre-saturation pulses outside the FOV or the imaging volume transfer magnetisation of flowing spins through 90° into the transverse plane (Fig. 8.2). Flowing spins, which then enter the imaging field, receive an additional 90° RF pulse within the imaging volume. The magnetisation of flowing spins is therefore flipped an additional 90° to 180°. Signal saturation from flowing spins occurs because no time is allowed for recovery of magnetisation. Given that flowing blood in vessels should appear black, persistent signal within vessel lumen after the application of saturation pulses indicates either slow flow, clot or vascular occlusion.

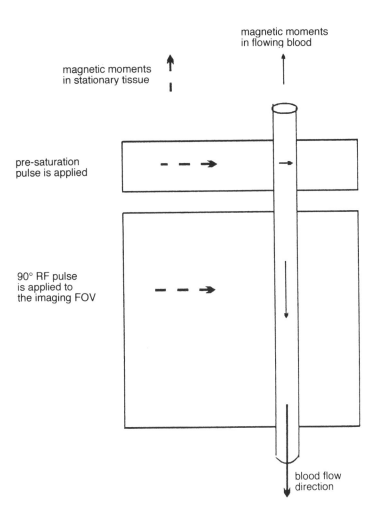

magnetic moments
in flowing blood

magnetic moments
in stationary tissue

pre-saturation
pulse is applied

90° RF pulse
is applied to
the imaging FOV

blood flow
direction

Fig. 8.2 Pre-saturation to
produce black blood.

Bright blood imaging

In addition to making the vessels appear black, vascular structures can also
be visualised by making them bright. Several techniques can be used to
enhance the signal from flowing blood including gradient echo imaging
and/or gradient moment rephasing and/or contrast enhancement. In
gradient echo imaging flowing spins are refocused by the rephasing
gradient and hence patent vessels appear bright on the image. As a result
this technique can be referred to as *bright blood imaging* (Fig. 8.3) and
can be further improved by the application of an imaging option known as
gradient moment rephasing (see Chapter 6). Gradient moment rephasing
is a first order velocity compensation technique used to visualise slow
moving protons with constant velocity. Protons in venous blood or CSF
are put into phase with the stationary protons, so that intra-voxel
dephasing is reduced. Gradient moment rephasing complements flow by

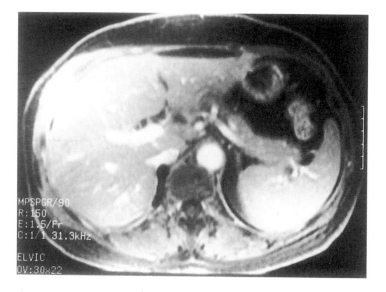

Fig. 8.3 This axial image of the liver was acquired with a gradient echo sequence. Note the high signal intensity in the abdominal vessels. Contrast enhancement was used to enhance signal in flowing vessels.

making vessels containing slow flowing spins appear bright, so enhancing the signal from blood and CSF.

Gradient moment rephasing is widely used in the chest and abdomen, brain, extremities and for the myelographic effect of CSF in T2 weighted images of the spine. There are however several trade-offs for using gradient moment rephasing. One such trade off is that it requires a longer minimum TE due to the use of additional gradients, and results in a reduction in the number of slices available. Another trade off is that gradient moment rephasing is not particularly effective on rapid flow in the chest or abdomen, however it is helpful for the visualisation of slow flow found in these areas.

LEARNING POINT

Pre-saturation can be used on both spin echo and gradient echo pulse sequences and in some instances it is appropriate to use both pre-saturation and gradient moment rephasing in the same sequence.

Another technique to enhance the signal from flowing blood is the administration of contrast agents (see Chapter 11).

Magnetic resonance angiography (MRA)

A more sophisticated means of imaging the vascular system is with the use of a technique known as *magnetic resonance angiography (MRA)*. Vascular contrast is maximised by enhancing the signal from moving spins in flowing blood and/or suppressing the signal from stationary spins residing in tissue. When stationary spins are suppressed, the appearance of vasculature is enhanced by the increased signal from fresh spins which flow into the imaging volume and receive RF excitation for the first time (sometimes known as the in-flow effect). There are two methods available to suppress stationary spins. First, two acquisitions can be performed which treat stationary spins identically, but which differentiate moving spins and subtract them. Secondly, if a short TR that saturates spins within the imaging volume is used in combination with the in-flow effect, a high degree of vascular contrast can be achieved. At present, there are four basic MRA techniques which utilise different phenomena to increase the signal from flowing spins and can be used to evaluate the cardiovascular system non-invasively. These techniques include:

(1) Digital subtraction MR angiography (DS-MRA),
(2) Time of flight MR angiography (TOF-MRA),
(3) Phase contrast MR angiography (PC-MRA),
(4) Velocity encoding techniques.

In addition another more invasive technique is to introduce a bolus injection of contrast medium followed by a 3D T1 gradient echo sequence.

Digital subtraction MRA

Digital subtraction MRA has been compared to digital subtraction angiography as contrast is selectively produced for moving spins during two acquisitions. These are then subtracted to remove the signal from the stationary spins, leaving behind an image of only the moving spins. An early subtraction angiogram has been performed while gating to the cardiac cycle. An acquisition during systole (fast flow), was subtracted from an acquisition during diastole (slow flow). In this case, the stationary spins were subtracted out, visualising only the moving spins (and hence the vasculature) on the resultant image. Although this is an out-dated technique and not widely used, it does deserve a brief mention in that it laid the ground work for some of the techniques used today.

Time of flight MRA

Time of flight MRA (TOF-MRA) produces vascular contrast by manipulating the longitudinal magnetisation of the stationary spins. TOF-MRA uses an incoherent gradient echo pulse sequence in combination with gradient moment rephasing to enhance flow. In TOF-MRA, the TR is kept well below the T1 time of the stationary tissues so that T1 recovery is prevented. This beats down the stationary spins, whilst the in-flow effect from fully magnetised flowing fresh spins produces high vascular signal. However if the TR is too short, the flowing spins may be suppressed along with the stationary spins which reduces vascular contrast. TOF-MRA can be acquired in 2D or 3D. In 2D TOF-MRA, a flip angle of 45–60° in conjunction with a TR of 40–50 ms, is usually sufficient to maximise signal without suppressing the signal from flowing nuclei. Within this flip angle and TR range, saturation of flowing spins only occurs at flow velocities of approximately 3 cm/s or less. In addition, signal intensities in flowing spins may be increased by shortening their T1 times with the use of contrast enhancement agents (see Chapter 11).

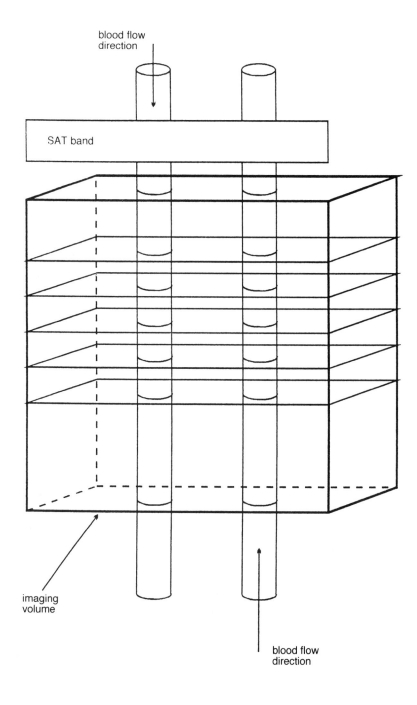

Fig. 8.4 Pre-saturation volume relative to the imaging stack.

To evaluate signals from arterial flow, it may be advisable to apply saturation pulses in the direction of venous flow. For example, to evaluate the carotid arteries in the neck, apply saturation pulses superior to the imaging volume to saturate the signal from inflowing venous blood (Fig. 8.4).

TOF-MRA is mostly sensitive to flow that comes perpendicularly into the FOV and the slice. Any flow which traverses the FOV can be saturated along with the stationary tissue if the flow velocities are slow relative to the TR. In addition, vessels with flow within the FOV may demonstrate some saturation of flowing spins since T1 recovery occurs over the time in which spins move down-stream in the imaging volume (Fig. 8.5). The result of these phenomena is a reduction in vascular signal.

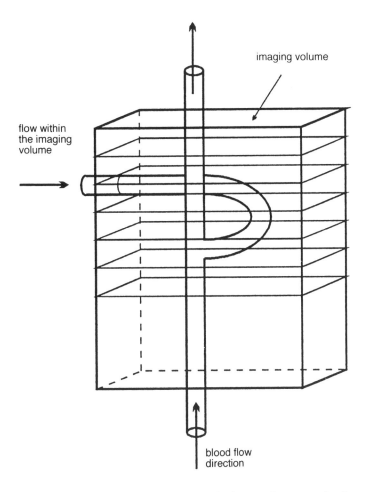

Fig. 8.5 Flow within the imaging volume.

Another disadvantage of TOF-MRA is high signal in some background tissues. Since TOF is acquired with an incoherent gradient echo sequence, tissues with short T1 times appear bright. Therefore despite saturation efforts, tissues with short T1 relaxation times can have a high signal on a TOF-MRA image. As a result of this phenomenon, high signal intensity can be seen for example in the orbit, caused by the short T1 of retro-orbital fat. This can be minimised by choosing a TE so that to a certain extent the signals from fat and water are out of phase with each other, and therefore cancel each other out. The TE should however be kept relatively short, to minimise intra-voxel dephasing and subsequent phase ghosting and signal loss. Another remedy for this high signal has been offered by several manufacturers who have included magnetisation transfer coherence (MTC) techniques (see Chapter 4) in TOF-MRA pulse sequences. Both solutions should help to minimise unwanted background signals. In addition blood components with a short T1 recovery time such as methaemaglobin, also appear bright on TOF-MRA. Therefore, there can be a problem in distinguishing sub-acute haemorrhage from flowing blood on TOF-MRA images.

2D versus 3D TOF-MRA

TOF-MRA can be acquired in either 2D (slice by slice) or 3D (volume) acquisition modes. In general, 3D volume imaging offers high SNR and thin contiguous slices for good resolution. However, as TOF-MRA is sensitive to flow coming into the FOV or the imaging volume, spins in vessels with slow flow can be saturated in volume imaging. For this reason, 3D TOF should be used in areas of high velocity flow (intra-cranial applications), and for high resolution to visualise small vessels (Fig. 8.6). 2D TOF is optimal in areas of slower velocity flow (carotids, peripheral vascular, and the venous systems) and when a large area of coverage is required. In 3D techniques, there is a higher risk of saturating signals from spins within the volume.

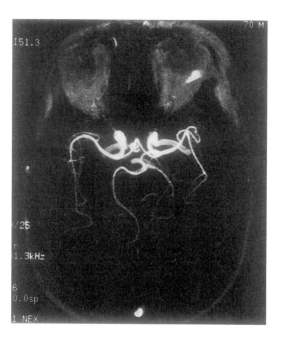

Fig. 8.6 This axial collapsed image of the brain was acquired with a 3D TOF-MRA. Note that small peripheral vessels are visualised with this technique.

Parameters and clinical suggestions for TOF-MRA

The carotid bifurcation, the peripheral circulation and cortical venous mapping can be imaged with 2D TOF-MRA. The parameters used for 2D TOF-MRA vary with manufacturer but generally the following should optimise image quality:

(1) TR 45 ms,
(2) minimum allowable TE,
(3) flip angles approximately 60°.

The selection of a short TR and medium flip angles allows for saturation of stationary nuclei but the moving spins coming into the slice remain fresh, and so vascular image contrast is maximised. The short TE reduces phase ghosting and susceptibility artefacts found on MR images acquired with gradient echo. Gradient moment rephasing, in conjunction with saturation pulses to suppress signals from areas of undesired flow, should be used to enhance vascular contrast relative to stationary tissue. Axial slice planes with slice thicknesses ranging from 1.5 mm (for the carotids and cortical venous structures) to 2.9 mm (for the peripheral vascular structures) should suffice.

TOF-MRA advantages

- Sensitive to T1 effects (short T1 tissues are bright. Contrast may be given for additional enhancement).
- Reasonable imaging times (approximately 5 min depending on parameters).
- Sensitive to slow flow.
- Reduced sensitivity to intra-voxel dephasing.

TOF-MRA disadvantages

- Sensitive to T1 effects (short T1 tissues are bright so that haemorrhagic lesions may mimic vessels).
- Saturation of in-plane flow (any flow within the FOV or volume of tissue can be saturated along with background tissue).
- Enhancement is limited to either flow entering the FOV or very high velocity flow.

2D TOF-MRA advantages

- Large area of coverage
- Sensitive to slow flow
- Sensitive to T1 effects

2D TOF-MRA disadvantages

- Lower resolution
- Saturation of in-plane flow
- Venetian blind artefact (occurs as respiration and patient motion moves tissue in and out of the slice that is being suppressed)

3D TOF-MRA advantages

- High resolution for small vessels
- Sensitive to T1 effects

3D TOF-MRA disadvantages

- Saturation of in-plane flow
- Small area of coverage

Overcoming the disadvantages of TOF-MRA

Therer are a number of ways of overcoming the limitations of TOF-MRA for both 2D and 3D acquisitions. These are listed above and there are several imaging options and protocol modifications that compensate for these pitfalls.

To overcome the susceptibility artefacts that are present on any gradient echo sequence, including MRA, short TEs and small voxel volumes should be utilised. In general, longer TEs permit more dephasing and therefore a TE of less than 4 ms minimises this artefact. The larger the voxel, the more intra-voxel dephasing and therefore small FOVs, thin slices and fine matrices will reduce this effect.

Poor background suppression can be corrected by either using TEs that acquire data when fat and water are out of phase or by implementing magnetisation transfer techniques. Out of phase images minimise the signal from tissues, such as fat, that have a short T1 relaxation time (see Chapter 7). MTC suppresses signal from macromolecules in fat and grey and white matter. As a result of improved background suppression, smaller peripheral vessels may be visualised (see Chapter 4).

Suppression of in-plane vascular signal, especially in 3D acquisitions, can be overcome by the utilisation of ramped RF pulses and via the administration of contrast media. Ramped RF pulses set flip angles across a 3D acquisition so that the flip angle increases across the volume of the slab. As a result, signal from spins that have flowed across the volume of tissue still produce signal at the end of the imaging volume. The administration of intravenous contrast agents also enhances signal from blood that might have otherwise been suppressed.

Motion artefacts can arise from a number of sources including respiration and pulsatile blood flow. Respiratory motion artefacts, known as Venetian blind artefacts, can be minimised by reducing respiration via breath-hold techniques. Pulsation artefacts can be reduced by timing the acquisition to the cardiac cycle. This technique is known as gating and will be discussed later in the chapter.

To overcome the limited coverage provided by 3D TOF-MRA, one can either acquire images in another plane or combine a number of 3D acquisitions in a technique known as MOTSA. MOTSA is Multiple Overlapping Thin Section Angiography. It combines a number of high resolution 3D acquisitions to produce an image that has good resolution and a large area of coverage.

A simpler approach would be to acquire images in the plane that best covers the anatomy. For example, to cover adequately the ascending and descending aortic arch the sagittal plane is optimal, whereas the coronal plane is better for the renal arteries and aorta. The problem with this strategy is that it is prone to in-plane flow. To overcome this a combination of 3D imaging with contrast enhancement, with rapid dynamic imaging may be used. Furthermore, to overcome small coverage, images can be acquired in the desired plane for adequate coverage. Figs 8.7 to 8.9 demonstrate different TOF-MRA techniques.

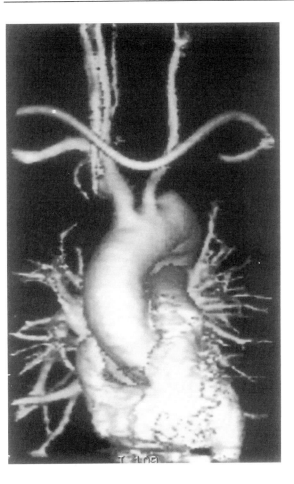 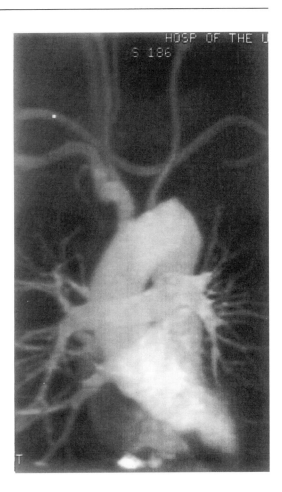

Fig. 8.7 These MRA images were acquired with a 3D gradient echo after dynamic contrast injection and then post-processed using MIP (left) and shaded surface display (right). The images were acquired in the sagittal plane to look at the ascending aorta, the arch and the descending aorta (the candy cane shot). The same technique can be used to visualise abdominal vessels in the coronal plane.

MRA image reformation

The manner in which the data from MRA images is reformatted, plays a large part in determining the way in which vascular anatomy is perceived in the images. One method for reformatting TOF-MRA image data, uses a technique known as *maximum pixel intensity (MIP)*. In this technique, a projection ray is passed through the volume of data so that this data is projected on to a two-dimensional plane. There is a mathematical correlation between each pixel in the projection image and the pixels along each line of the volume data. A projection pixel is assigned the maximum intensity found along the projection ray passing through the volume data. Subsequent intensities detected by the ray are assigned lesser signal intensities. This process is repeated at different projection angles and the resultant images are then combined to give a three-dimensional perception of vascular structures. This technique is known as MIP with a

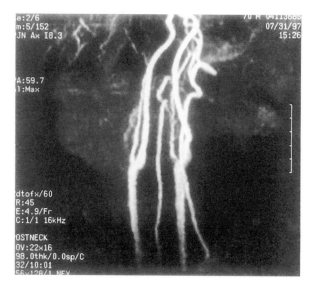

Fig. 8.8 This TOF image was acquired with 2D acquisition. Note the large coverage from the origins of the neck vessels to the circle of Willis.

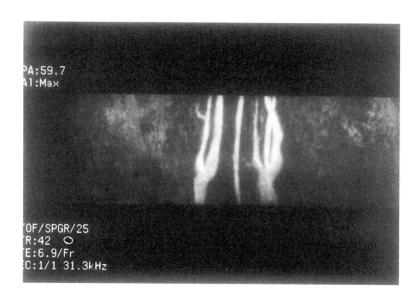

Fig. 8.9 This TOF-MRA was acquired in 3D acquisition. Note the high resolution of the carotid bifurcations.

ray trace algorithm or *depth queuing*. With the use of a ray trace algorithm, the image is viewed so that the vascular anatomy nearest to the observer appears brighter than that which is furthest away. As a result, the viewer has a perception of the depth of the image data (Fig. 8.10).

Another method of reformatting MRA images is with a Shaded Surface Display (SSD). This technique reformats image data as though a light is shone onto structures (as opposed to MIP which is similar to a light shining through structures). This results in a 3D appearance of the vasculature (Fig. 8.7).

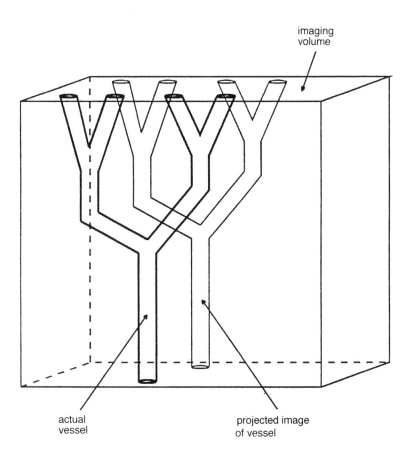

imaging
volume

actual
vessel

projected image
of vessel

Fig. 8.10 MIP reformatting.

Phase contrast MRA

Phase contrast MRA utilises the velocity differences, and hence the phase shifts in moving spins, to provide image contrast in flowing vessels. The variation in phase originates from physiological conditions such as systolic and diastolic velocity changes. Phase shifts can also be generated in the pulse sequence by phase encoding the velocity of flow with the use of a bipolar (two lobes that are equal in strength, one negative one positive) gradient. In this method, phase shift is introduced selectively for moving spins with the use of magnetic field gradients. This technique is known as phase contrast magnetic resonance angiography (PC-MRA). PC-MRA is sensitive to flow within, as well as that coming perpendicularly into the FOV and the slice (Fig. 8.11).

Immediately after the RF, excitation pulse spins are in phase (time A). In PC-MRA a gradient of a given strength is applied to both stationary and flowing spins. Although phase shifts occur in both stationary and flowing spins, these shifts occur at different rates. During initial application of the first bipolar gradient (time B), there is a shift of phases of stationary spins (left) and flowing spins (right). After the second part of the application of the first bipolar gradient (time C), the stationary spins (left) return to their

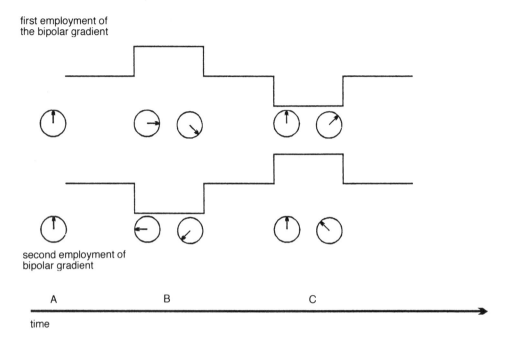

first employment of
the bipolar gradient

second employment of
bipolar gradient

A   B   C

time

Fig. 8.11 Bipolar gradients to produce phase contrast.

initial phase (time A), but those of moving spins (right) acquire some phase.

The bipolar gradient is then applied with opposite polarity or direction but at the same strength or amplitude so that the same variants occur, but in the opposite direction. PC-MRA then subtracts the two acquisitions so that the signals from stationary spins are subtracted out leaving only the signals from flowing spins. The combination of PC-MRA acquisitions results in what are known as magnitude and phase images. The unsubtracted combinations of flow sensitised image data are known as magnitude images, whereas the subtracted combinations are called phase images.

Flow encoding axes

Sensitisation to flow is obtained along the direction of the applied bipolar gradient. If the bipolar gradient pulses are applied along the Z-axis, phase shifts are induced in flow that occurs along this axis, so sensitising the PC-MRA to flow which runs from head to foot. Since flow can occur in other directions, bipolar gradients are applied in all three dimensions and in doing so, sensitise flow in all three directions X, Y, and Z (Fig. 8.12). These are known as flow encoding axes. However, an increase in the number of flow encoding axes also increases the imaging time.

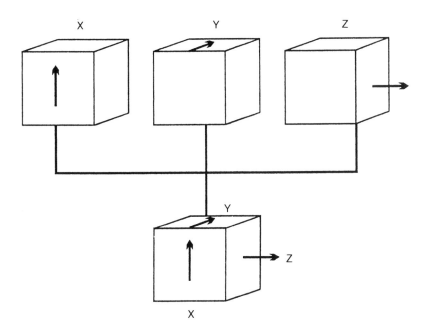

Fig. 8.12   Flow encoding axes.

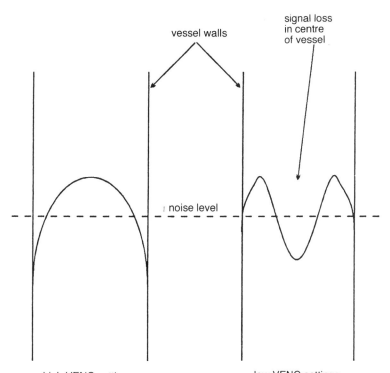

Fig. 8.13   VENC settings.

Velocity encoding (VENC)

PC-MRA can also be sensitised to flow velocity. Velocity encoding technique (VENC) compensates for projected flow velocity within vessels by controlling the amplitude or strength, of the bipolar gradient. If the VENC selected is lower than the velocity within the vessel, aliasing can occur. This results in low signal intensity in the centre of the vessel, but better delineation of the vessel wall itself. It occurs because high velocity laminar flow is found in the centre of the vessel, the signal from which is aliased or mismapped out of the vessel lumen. However, there is better delineation of the vessel wall above background noise levels. Conversely, with high VENC settings, intra-luminal signal is improved, but vessel wall delineation is compromised (Fig. 8.13).

2D and 3D PC-MRA

PC-MRA can be acquired with the use of either 2D or 3D acquisition strategies. Two dimensional techniques provide acceptable imaging times (1 to 3 min) and flow direction information. If a 2D PC-MRA acquisition has been flow encoded from superior to inferior, flow from the head appears white, whereas flow from the feet appears black. 2D acquisitions, however, sometimes cannot be reformatted and viewed in other imaging planes. As in clinical imaging, 3D offers SNR and spatial resolution superior to 2D imaging strategies, and the ability to reformat in a number of imaging planes retrospectively. The trade-off however is that in 3D PC-MRA, imaging time increases with the TR, NEX, the number of phase encoding steps, the number of slices and the number of flow encoding axes selected. For this reason, scan times can approach 15 min or more.

Parameters and clinical suggestions for PC-MRA

PC-MRA can be used effectively in the evaluation of arteriovenous malformations, aneurysms, venous occlusions, congenital abnormalities and traumatic intra-cranial vascular injuries. 3D volume acquisitions can be used to evaluate intra-cranial vasculature. Suggested parameters are:

28 slices volume, 1 mm slice thickness
flip angle 20° (60 slice volume flip angle reduced to 15°)
TR less than or equal to 25 ms
VENC 40–60 cm/s
flow encoding in all directions

2D techniques offer more acceptable imaging times of approximately 1 to 3 min. For intra-cranial applications of 2D PC-MRA suggested parameters are:

TR 18–20 ms
flip angle 20°
slices thickness 20–60 mm

VENCs
>20–30 cm/s for venous flow
>40–60 cm/s for higher velocity with some aliasing
>60–80 cm/s to determine velocity and flow direction

For carotids 2D PC-MRA parameters include:

flip angles 20°–30°

TR 20 ms

VENCs
>40–60 cm/s for better morphology with aliasing
>60–80 cm/s for quantitative velocity and directional information

Advantages of PC-MRA

- Sensitivity to a variety of vascular velocities
- Sensitivity to flow within the FOV
- Reduced intra-voxel dephasing
- Increased background suppression
- Magnitude and phase images.

Disadvantages of PC-MRA

- Long imaging times with 3D
- More sensitive to turbulence.

Velocity encoding techniques

Velocity encoding techniques are designed to evaluate flow velocity and direction providing information similar to Doppler ultrasound. The projection plane is located at right angles to the excitation plane. The location of vascular plugs on the projection plane shows flow direction, and length of the projection defines the velocity of flow (Fig. 8.14).

Magnetic resonance angiography summary

The information provided by PC and TOF-MRA differs from that of conventional contrast-angiography as MRA produces a flow sensitive image, rather than a morphological image. Consequently, clinical situations which require haemodynamic information are more suited to MRA than those requiring fine anatomic detail. Using MRA, laminar flow can be clearly imaged. However, as turbulent flow contains dispersion velocities which result in dephasing within a voxel, a loss of signal intensity results. In many respects, information provided by MRA is a combination of the flow information obtained in a Doppler ultrasound examination, and the morphological information contained in conventional contrast

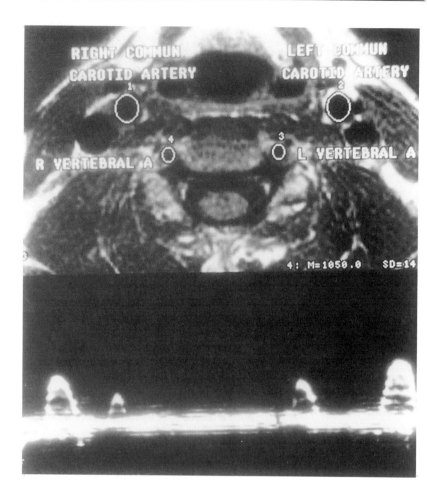

Fig. 8.14 Axial T1 weighted image of the neck (above) with the velocity encoded image (below). The size of the plugs determines velocity and the location shows direction of blood flow.

angiography. This is especially true when PC and TOF-MRA are used in combination with velocity encoding techniques (Fig. 8.15).

Perfusion and diffusion imaging

It appears that perfusion and diffusion imaging represents the next step, after MRI and MRA in non-invasive tissue characterisation. Diffusion is the translational motion of water molecules in any direction, but distinct from those rotations responsible for T1 recovery and T2 decay. Diffusion imaging uses balanced gradients to preserve signal intensity in stationary spins, but also to reduce the signal intensity of diffusing water protons. In water diffusion is usually isotropic, but in tissue which restricts diffusion it occurs anisotropically (see Chapter 12).

Perfusion is micro-circulation or the delivery of blood to tissues. Perfusion imaging is the measurement of blood volume in these areas. This measurement however is complicated, because less than 5% of tissue

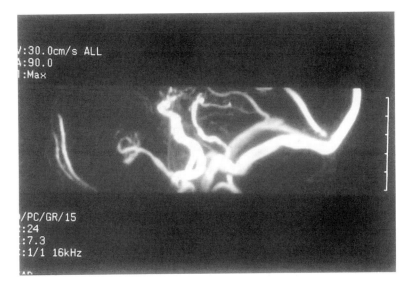

Fig. 8.15(a) This axial image of the brain was acquired with a 3D PC-MRA and projected in the sagittal plane. Parameters were chosen to visualise the venous flow in the transverse sinus as well as arterial flow up to the circle of Willis. Note that the background suppression is better than with TOF-MRA.

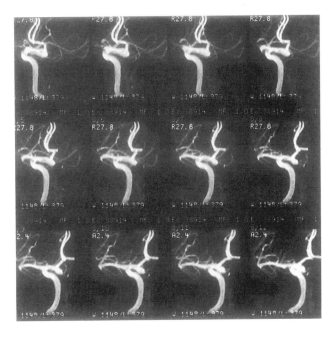

Fig. 8.15(b) This series of images represents post-processing for MRA whereby the vessel of interest is segmented out from the other vessels and projected in a number of obliquities. Note that the smaller vessels are visualised with depth on this MIP display as nearer vessels appear bright and vessels at the back appear dark.

protons are intra-vascular. To measure perfusion either stationary spins can be suppressed, or signal intensity in perfusing spins increased. This can be achieved by either employing motion sensitive gradients, additionally or introducing enhancement agents (see Chapter 12).

Vascular imaging techniques have now been described in general. To image the heart and great vessels specifically, the motion of these organs during cardiac activity must be compensated for, if good quality images are to be obtained. This is achieved using a technique known as cardiac gating.

Cardiac gating

Cardiac gating is a method that reduces the phase mismapping produced as a result of heart motion and pulsatile blood flow. It uses the electrical signal of the heart, or the mechanical flow of the vascular bed, to trigger each pulse sequence. Two methods are used:

(1) electrocardiogram (ECG, EKG) gating; uses electrodes and lead wires placed on to the patient's chest to detect the electrical activity of the heart,
(2) peripheral gating; uses a photo-sensor placed on the patient's finger to detect a pulse in the capillary bed.

The ECG

The ECG is acquired by measuring the voltage difference between two electrodes attached to the patient's chest. Most systems colour code the electrodes so that they can be placed correctly. The red and the white electrodes are usually placed across the heart, as these measure the voltage difference between two points. The green electrode is the ground, and should be placed as near to (but not touching), either the red or the white electrode.

The ECG consists of:

(1) a P wave that represents atrial systole (contraction),
(2) a QRS complex that represents ventricular systole,
(3) a T wave that represents ventricular diastole (relaxation).

The peak of the R wave is used to trigger each pulse sequence because electrically, it has the greatest amplitude (Fig. 8.16).

The effective TR

As cardiac gating uses each R wave to trigger the pulse sequence, the TR depends entirely on the time interval between each R wave. This is called

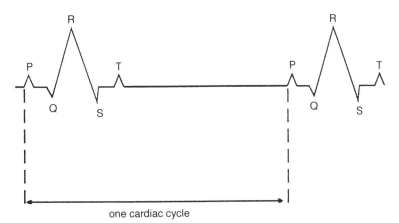

Fig. 8.16 The ECG.

one cardiac cycle

the R to R interval and is controlled by the patient's heart rate (Fig. 8.17). If a patient has a fast rate, the RR interval is shorter, than if the patient has a slow heart rate. The TR, and therefore the image weighting and number of slices, depends totally on the heart rate. The TR is now termed 'effective' as the heart rate is not perfectly constant and varies from one heart beat to another.

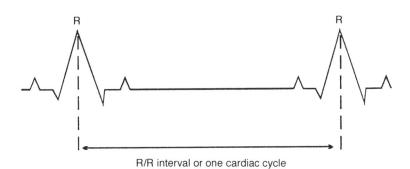

Fig. 8.17 The R to R interval.

R/R interval or one cardiac cycle

For example, if the heart rate is 60 beats per minute then:

$$R \text{ to } R \text{ interval} = 60\,000 \text{ ms}/60 = 1000 \text{ ms}.$$

(There are 60 seconds per minute and 1000 milliseconds per second or 1 heartbeat every second.)

If the patient's heart rate is 120 beats per minute then:

$$R \text{ to } R \text{ interval is } 500 \text{ ms}$$

This seems to be very restrictive in terms of weighting and slice number. To a certain extent this is true, in that there is no control of the R to R interval itself. In some patients the effective TR is 500 ms, and in others the TR is over 1000 ms which reduces the T1 weighting considerably.

This has to be tolerated when using gating techniques, as a penalty for producing images with reduced cardiac motion artefact. Figure 8.18 shows the T1 weighted axial image of the heart using ECG gating.

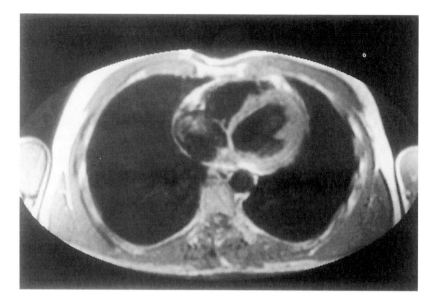

Fig. 8.18 This axial image of the chest was acquired with spin echo and cardiac gating. With prospective gating employed, the visualisation of the cardiac chambers and great vessels of the chest are made possible. As this is a spin echo sequence, flowing blood appears dark.

Obtaining T2 weighted images can be more troublesome, but most systems use a method whereby every second or third R wave can be used as a trigger. In this way, the effective TR is lengthened so that saturation (and therefore T1 weighting) does not prevail, and proton density (short TE), and T2 (long TE) images can be obtained.

For example, if the R to R interval is 1000 ms:

1 R to R selected effective TR = 1000 ms
2 R to R selected effective TR = 2000 ms
3 R to R selected effective TR = 3000 ms

To achieve T1 weighting, use each R wave to trigger each pulse sequence. This gives an effective TR of 600–1000 ms, depending on the patient's heart rate. For proton density and T2 weighting, use every second or third R wave to trigger, as this gives an effective TR of 2000–3000 ms, depending on the patient's heart rate.

Slice acquisition

The slices are acquired during the effective TR in the same way as in conventional imaging. Phase encoding data from each slice is acquired during the R to R interval. During the next interval data from another phase encoding step is acquired (Fig. 8.19). This is repeated until the acquisition of data (or all the phase encoding steps) for each slice is

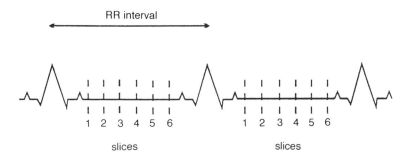

Fig. 8.19 Slice acquisition during the R to R interval.

complete. Data from each slice is always acquired when the heart is at the same phase of cardiac activity. In other words, slice 1 is always acquired when the heart is at a certain position in its cycle, and so are slices 2, 3, etc. In this way, the motion artefact of each slice is reduced.

This of course, only applies if the patient's heart rate remains constant throughout the scan. If the rate changes at all, data is obtained at different times during the cardiac cycle, and the images contain a great deal of artefact. Most patients' heart rates do not remain constant, but fluctuate due to anxiety or the gradient noise during the sequence. In order to compensate for this, certain safeguards are built into the effective TR so that gating is more efficient. These safeguards occur in the form of waiting periods around each R wave. These waiting periods are termed in many different ways, but basically there is a waiting period just before each R wave, and one just after. Many imaging systems automatically build these waiting periods into the pulse sequences. Others provide these as user-selectable parameters.

The trigger window

The waiting period before each R wave is often called the *trigger window*. This is a time delay, usually expressed as a percentage of the total R to R interval, where the system stops scanning and waits for the next R wave (Fig. 8.20).

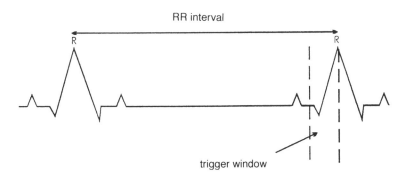

Fig. 8.20 The trigger window.

This delay allows for the fact that the patient's heart rate may increase during the scan, moving the R wave nearer to the beginning of the window. If the system has stopped scanning and is waiting for the next R wave, it triggers the pulse sequence, regardless of whether the R wave is occurring sooner than expected. If the heart rate speeds up even more, so that the R wave occurs while the system is still acquiring data, the R wave is missed and the effective TR suddenly lengthens (Fig. 8.21).

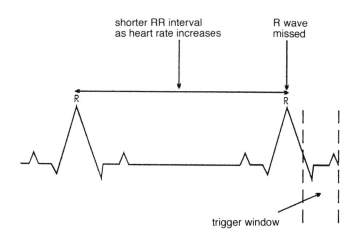

Fig. 8.21 A missed R wave as the heart rate increases.

If the heart rate slows down, the R wave moves further away from the beginning of the window, but the system is still waiting to trigger the scan and does so when it detects the next R wave. The effective TR is lengthened but the R wave is not missed (Fig. 8.22).

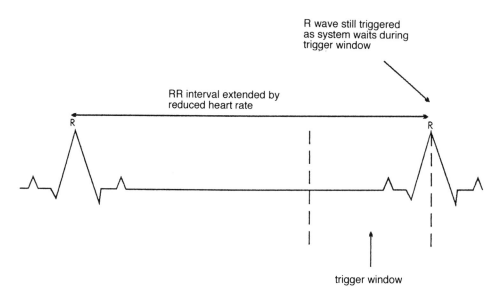

Fig. 8.22 The R wave is not missed as the heart rate decreases.

The trigger window is usually expressed as a percentage of the R to R interval. Clearly, the correct window must be selected so that any increase in the heart rate is compensated for. Selecting a very large window however, reduces the amount of time available to acquire slices and so a balance is required. In practice, most patient's heart rate varies by about 10% during the scan, so selecting a window of about 10 to 20% compensates adequately for any variations in the heart rate and still allows a reasonable number of slices to be acquired (Fig. 8.23).

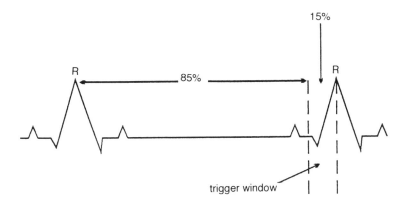

Fig. 8.23 What would the trigger window be if the RR interval was 1000 ms?

The trigger delay

The waiting period after each R wave is often termed the delay after trigger. There is always a slight hardware delay between the system detecting the R wave and transmitting RF to excite the first slice. This is usually in the order of a few ms. This period can often be extended however, to delay the acquisition of the slices until the heart is in diastole and is therefore relatively still (Fig. 8.24).

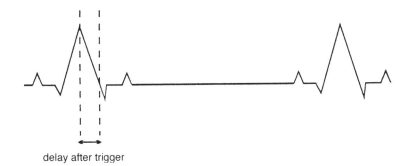

Fig. 8.24 The delay after trigger.

The available imaging time

The available imaging time is the time actually available to acquire slices. It is defined as the effective TR minus the trigger window and the delay after trigger.

Available imaging time = RR interval – (trigger window + trigger delay)

If the RR interval is 1000 ms, the trigger window 10% and the trigger delay 100 ms the time available to acquire the data is

$$1000 - 100 - 100 = 800 \text{ ms}$$

The available imaging time is not the effective TR. The effective TR is the time between the excitation of slice 1 in the first R to R interval, to its excitation in the second R to R interval. The available imaging time is purely the time allowed to collect data, and governs the number of slices that can be obtained (Fig. 8.25).

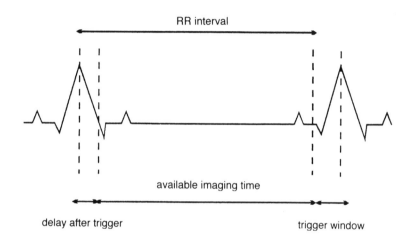

Fig. 8.25 The available imaging time.

Peripheral gating

Peripheral gating works in exactly the same way as ECG gating. A photo-sensor attached to the patient's finger, detects the increase in blood volume in the capillary bed during systole. This in turn, affects the amount of light reflected back to the sensor and a wave form is obtained. The peaks of the waves are now termed the R waves, but these actually represent the peripheral pulse that occurs approximately 250 ms after the R wave of the ECG. The trigger window, trigger delay and available imaging time still apply.

Parameters used in gating

T1 weighting
    Short TE
     1 R to R interval
PD/T2 weighting
    Short TE (PD)/long TE (T2)
     2 or 3 R to R intervals

Safety aspects of gating

The electrodes used in gating are attached to cables that are conductors and are therefore capable of carrying relatively high currents. The cables lie within the high intensity region of the gradient field during the scan. As a result, currents may be induced in the cables which can potentially store and transfer heat to the patient. It is therefore possible to burn or blister the patient, if strict safety rules are not adhered to.

Always check the cables and electrodes for damage. If they are frayed or splitting do not use them under any circumstances. When positioning the cables, avoid looping or crossing them over. The point of cross-over creates extra heat that could burn through the insulating material of the cable. When positioning the patient within the bore of the magnet, make sure that the cables do not touch either the patient or the bore of the magnet. Running the cables down the centre of the patient avoids contact with the bore, and placing pads between the cables and the patient prevents possible injury.

The uses of gating

Gating is useful when imaging any area that contains pulsatile flow, or the heart itself. This includes the chest and great vessels, the abdomen, the spinal cord (CSF pulsations) and the brain. Virtually any area where pulsatile motion degrades the image lends itself to gating of some sort. The decision to use ECG or peripheral gating is often difficult. ECG gating is more time consuming because of the electrode placement, and because arrhythmias can alter the ECG to such an extent that the system cannot detect an adequate R wave. These difficulties are usually not present with peripheral gating, but this is not adequate when imaging the heart itself. Generally, peripheral gating is adequate for the brain, spine and vessels away from the heart. ECG gating should be used for the heart itself.

Gating is a rather lengthy process as the time of the scan is determined (amongst other things), by the patient's heart rate. A patient with bradycardia is not welcomed in an MRI suite! For this reason, many sites reserve gating only for chest imaging.

- ECG gating reduces motion artefact so that anatomy can be demonstrated well.
- It requires electrode and lead placement on the patient.
- Usually there is no control over the TR, weighting or slice number when using gating.
- Gating is relatively time consuming especially if the heart rate is slow.

Pseudo-gating

This is a very simple method of gating that involves selecting a TR that matches the R to R interval. ECG and peripheral gating is not employed but instead, the patient's heart rate is measured before the examination by taking the pulse. The R to R interval is then calculated (60 000/heart rate in ms) and the TR corresponding to this is selected. As long as the heart rate does not significantly change during the examination, data from each slice is acquired at exactly the same time during the cardiac cycle as in conventional gating. This technique may be useful when conventional gating fails due to a poor ECG signal or low peripheral pulse. However to be most effective, the heart rate must remain unaltered during the examination.

Gating is essential when studying the anatomy of the heart and great vessels. However a study of heart function, requires multiple images acquired at multiple phases of the cardiac cycle. This can be achieved using multi-phase imaging or cine.

Multi-phase cardiac imaging

In multi-phase cardiac imaging, a spin-echo pulse sequence is used with slices acquired at precise phases of the cardiac cycle. This technique can be performed with either single-slice or multi-slice acquisition techniques. In multi-slice acquisition, the first slice location is acquired in each of four phases of the cardiac cycle. This is then repeated at the other slice locations. All the images acquired at each slice location can be placed in a 'loop' so that they may be viewed rapidly one after the other. In this way, cardiac motion can be visualised and cardiac function evaluated. One drawback is that the imaging time increases with the number of slice locations and/or phases imaged.

Cine

Cine is a method of collecting data continuously throughout the cardiac cycle, so that data from each slice is acquired at different points during the cycle. This data can then be reconstructed into a loop, so that each slice demonstrates cardiac function. Cine is usually performed during a gradient echo sequence. ECG or peripheral gating must be used, but data collection is continuous not triggered. The ECG is purely used to determine the phase of the cardiac cycle, so that after the acquisition the system can sort the data and reconstruct the images across the whole of the cardiac cycle (Fig. 8.26).

Parameters used in cine

It is necessary to obtain good contrast between the vessel to be imaged with cine and the surrounding tissue. T2* weighted coherent gradient echo sequences are used, so that blood or CSF appears bright. Gradient echo sequences are flow sensitive, because gradient reversal is not slice

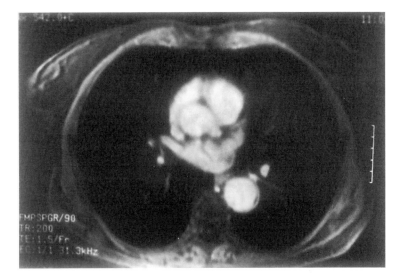

Fig. 8.26 This axial image of the chest was acquired with gradient echo and cine. With retrospective gating employed, and multiple phases of the heart acquired, the evaluation of cardiac function is possible. Since this is a gradient echo sequence, flowing blood appears bright.

selective (as in spin echo). Therefore, a flowing nucleus produces signal after gradient rephasing, regardless of its slice location during excitation (see Chapter 6). Using a pulse sequence that employs coherent transverse magnetisation in conjunction with the steady state, maximises $T2^*$ weighting (GRASS, FFE, FISP). A short TR (in the order of 40 ms) in conjunction with flip angles of 30°–45° should be selected to maintain the steady state. Using a short TR ensures that the stationary spins within the slice become saturated or beaten down by rapid successive RF pulses, whereas the flowing spins enter the slices relatively fresh. This saturates the background stationary tissue and enhances the brightness of the flowing nuclei. The TE should be relatively long to enhance $T2^*$ weighting (about 20 ms), and the use of gradient moment rephasing maximises contrast even further. Some systems also permit cine acquisitions with incoherent gradient echo sequences. These can be used to give T1 weighted cine images. To optimise vascular contrast however use:

- coherent gradient echo sequences,
- a TR of less than 50 ms/flip angles 30°–45° (to maintain the steady state and saturate stationary nuclei),
- TE 15–25 ms to maximise $T2^*$,
- gradient moment rephasing to enhance bright blood.

Data collection

The data is collected from each slice at a certain interval across the cardiac cycle. The R to R interval and the effective TR for each slice determine how many times this data can be collected during each cardiac cycle. Data is collected at data points during the cycle. In addition, the number of phases of the cardiac cycle required to make up the cine loop can be selected. For example, if 16 phases are selected each slice must demonstrate 16 different positions of the heart in one cardiac cycle (compared with 4 phases in multi-phase imaging). This is analogous to frames per second, but in cine it refers to the number of phases per cardiac cycle.

In order to do this accurately, the collection of data must correlate as much as possible to each cardiac phase (Fig. 8.27). Each data point must coincide with each cardiac phase. If the system cannot match the data points and the phases, it takes some data from one point and some from another, to form the image at a certain phase position. Under these circumstances, cine does not work efficiently (Fig. 8.28).

phases

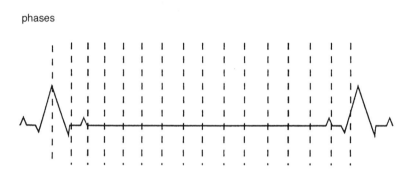

Fig. 8.27 Data acquisition in cine imaging.

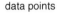

data points

phases

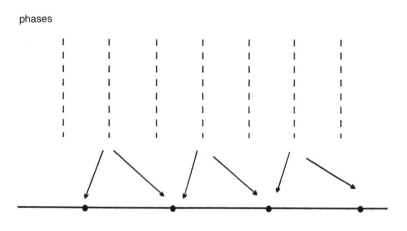

Fig. 8.28 Mismatching of data points and phases.

data points

In practice, it is therefore important to calculate how many data points the system can collect for a given R to R interval, and ensure that the number of phases selected does not exceed this. The number of data points can be calculated by dividing the R to R interval by the effective TR. In cine, the effective TR for each slice is the TR selected multiplied by the number of slices prescribed.

For example, if a TR of 40 ms is selected and two slices are prescribed, the effective TR is 80 ms.

The effective TR in cine is therefore very different from that used in gating, and the two should not be confused. In gating, the TR is not selectable as it is determined by the R to R interval. In cine although gating is used, the data is collected across the whole of the cardiac cycle and a TR is selectable. The ECG trace is purely used by the system to measure the cardiac cycle, not to trigger the pulse sequence. The effective TR of each slice in cine imaging, is the time between the collection of data for each slice. The number of data points collected is therefore determined by this, and the R to R interval of each cardiac cycle. If the effective TR is 80 ms and the R to R interval is 800 ms, 10 data points can be collected during each cardiac cycle. In order to cine efficiently, the number of cardiac phases reconstructed should not exceed 10 in this example.

The uses of cine

Cine is useful for dynamic imaging of vessels and CSF. For example, cine can evaluate aortic dissection and cardiac function. In the brain, it may be useful to demonstrate dynamically the flow of CSF in patients with hydrocephalus.

SPAMM

In addition to the classic cardiac imaging techniques there are new advances currently used in research. One of these techniques is known as *spatial modulation of magnetisation* (SPAMM). SPAMM modulates the magnetisation thus creating a saturation effect on the image. This effect can be seen on the image appearing as a cross-hatching of stripes. SPAMM is used in association with a multi-slice multi-phase acquisition and acquires data along the short axis of the left ventricle. In normal hearts, the stripes move along with the cardiac muscle. However in cases of infarction, the infarcted area does not contract along with the normal muscle, and can therefore be easily identified in relation to the stripes.

Therefore, cardiac and vascular imaging can be a useful tool in the evaluation of a whole host of clinical situations. However, there are many logistical drawbacks. Motion artefact is a constant problem and patient co-operation is essential. In addition, radiographer education is a funda-mental necessity if consistently diagnostic cardiac and vascular images are to be obtained. Recently, the quality and applications of cardiac MRI have increased with the use of EPI sequences (Chapter 12).

Questions

1. Vascular imaging can only be achieved with MRA techniques. True or false?

2. On spin echo images, flowing blood usually appears:
   (a) bright
   (b) dark
   (c) intermediate.

3. Gradient moment rephasing is applied to make flowing vessels appear:
   (a) bright
   (b) dark
   (c) intermediate.

4. TOF-MRA utilises a:
   (a) coherent gradient echo sequence
   (b) incoherent gradient echo sequence
   (c) coherent spin echo sequence
   (d) incoherent spin echo sequence.

5. Which of the following is best used to visualise small vessels:
   (a) 2D TOF?
   (b) 2D PC?
   (c) 3D TOF?
   (d) 3D PC?

6. Why do we use a trigger window in gating?

7. What is the available imaging time using these parameters?
   RR 800 ms
   trigger window 10% delay after trigger 4 m.

8. Indicate when you would use ECG, peripheral gating, or nothing when examining the following areas:
   (a) brain
   (b) knee
   (c) liver
   (d) mediastinum.

Chapter 9   Instrumentation and Equipment

Introduction

Several processes must be completed in order to produce magnetic resonance images. These processes include nuclear alignment, radio frequency excitation, spatial encoding and image formation. The hardware required to complete such processes includes:

(1) a magnet,
(2) a radio frequency source,
(3) an image processor,
(4) a computer system.

The magnet aligns the nuclei into low energy (parallel) and high energy (anti parallel) states. To maintain magnetic evenness or homogeneity, a shim system is necessary. A radio frequency (RF) source perturbs or excites nuclei. The RF system requires a transmitter and a receiver. Magnetic field gradients determine spatial locations of RF signals. The MR signal is changed to an understandable format from a FID into a spectrum by a series of mathematical equations known as Fourier transformations. This process occurs via the array processor. The host computer oversees the process and allows a means for operator interface with the system (Fig. 9.1). This chapter discusses magnetic resonance instrumentation in more detail. First however, magnetism and magnetic properties in general are described as this helps to understand different magnet types.

Magnetism

Like the mass and electrical charge of a particular substance, magnetism is a fundamental property of matter. All substances possess some form of magnetism. The degree of magnetism exhibited by any particular substance depends on the magnetic susceptibility of the atoms which

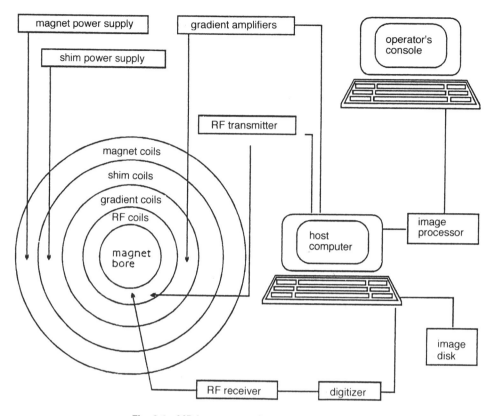

Fig. 9.1 MR instrumentation.

make up the substance. The magnetic susceptibility of a substance is the ability of external magnetic fields to effect the nuclei of a particular atom, and is related to the electron configurations of that atom. For example, the nucleus of an atom which is surrounded by paired electrons or an electron cloud, is more protected from and unaffected by, the external magnetic field. The nucleus of an atom with unpaired electrons however, is more exposed to the effects of the magnetic field. Depending on the nature of a substance's response to a magnetic field it can be classified as either paramagnetic, diamagnetic or ferromagnetic.

Paramagnetism

As the result of unpaired electrons within the atom, paramagnetic substances induce a small magnetic field about themselves known as the magnetic moment. With no external magnetic field these magnetic moments occur in a random pattern and thus cancel each other out. However in the presence of an external magnetic field, paramagnetic substances align with the direction of the field and so the magnetic

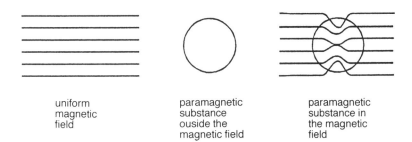

uniform
magnetic
field

paramagnetic
substance
ouside the
magnetic field

paramagnetic
substance in
the magnetic
field

Fig. 9.2 Paramagnetic properties.

moments add together (Fig. 9.2). Therefore paramagnetic substances affect external magnetic fields in a positive way, by attraction to the field resulting in a local increase in the magnetic field. One example of a paramagnetic substance is oxygen. Another is gadolinium chelates used as MR contrast agents.

Diamagnetism

With no external magnetic field present, diamagnetic substances, such as silver and copper, show no net magnetic moment. This is due to the fact that the electron currents caused by their motions add to zero. However when an external magnetic field is applied, diamagnetic substances show a small magnetic moment which opposes the applied field. Substances of this type are therefore not attracted to, but are slightly repelled by, the magnetic field. For this reason, diamagnetic substances have negative magnetic susceptibilities and show a slight decrease in magnetic field strength within the sample (Fig. 9.3). Examples of diamagnetic substances include inert gases, copper, sodium chloride, and sulphur.

Diamagnetic effects appear in all substances. However, in materials which possess both diamagnetic and paramagnetic properties, the positive paramagnetic effect is greater than the negative diamagnetic effect, and so the substance appears paramagnetic. The apparent magnetisation of an atom can be shown by the following equation

$$B = H_0 (1+x)$$

where B is the magnetic field and H_0 magnetic intensity.

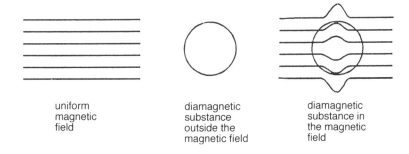

uniform
magnetic
field

diamagnetic
substance
outside the
magnetic field

diamagnetic
substance in
the magnetic
field

Fig. 9.3 Diamagnetic properties.

A substance is diamagnetic when x < 0. A substance is paramagnetic when x > 0.

Ferromagnetism

Ferromagnetic substances differ a great deal from diamagnetic and paramagnetic substances. When a ferromagnetic substance, such as iron, comes in contact with a magnetic field, the results are strong attraction and alignment. Objects made of substances of this type can become dangerous projectiles when inadvertently brought near a strong magnetic field. They retain their magnetisation even when the external magnetic field has been removed. Therefore, ferromagnetic substances remain magnetic, are permanently magnetised and subsequently become *permanent magnets*. The magnetic field in permanent magnets can be hundreds or even thousands of times greater than the applied external magnetic field (Fig. 9.4).

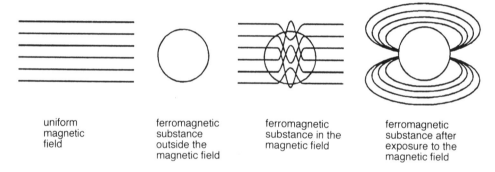

| uniform magnetic field | ferromagnetic substance outside the magnetic field | ferromagnetic substance in the magnetic field | ferromagnetic substance after exposure to the magnetic field |

Fig. 9.4 Ferromagnetic properties.

Permanent magnets are bipolar as they have two poles, north and south. The magnetic field exerted by a permanent magnet produces magnetic field lines or lines of force running from the magnetic south to the north poles of the magnet. The magnetic field of the earth also illustrates this phenomenon, which can be demonstrated with the use of a compass. The magnetic needle of the compass aligns with the lines of force of the earth and points toward the north pole. If the bar magnet is now bent in half, creating a horseshoe magnet, the lines of force still run from the south to the north poles of the magnet.

The strength of the magnetic field, expressed by the notation (B), (or in the case of more than one field, the primary field (B_0) and the secondary field (B_1), can be measured in one of three units; gauss (G), kilogauss (kG), and tesla (T). Gauss is a measure of low magnetic field strengths. For example, the strength of the earth's magnetic field is approximately 0.6 G. Tesla, on the other hand, is the unit used to measure higher magnetic field strengths. The three units of measurement can be compared with the use of the equation

$$1\,T = 10\,(kG) = 10\,000\,G$$

Most MR systems operate from as low as 0.3 T to as high as 2 T. Higher field strengths systems are used for research purposes. However, the strength of the magnetic field is not perfectly even across the entire field. The evenness within the magnetic field is termed *homogeneity*. Inhomogeneity within a particular magnetic field is expressed in an arbitrary unit known as parts per million (ppm). An inhomogeneity of 1 ppm in a 1 Tesla magnet yields a range in field strength from 10 000.00 to 10 000.01 G.

Now the various magnetic properties of matter have been described, the different types of magnet available are now explored. These are:

(1) permanent magnets,
(2) electromagnets (solenoidal and resistive),
(3) super conducting magnets

Permanent magnets

Since ferromagnetic substances retain their magnetism after being exposed to a magnetic field these substances are used in the production of a permanent magnet. Examples of substances used are iron, cobalt, and nickel. The most common material used to produce a permanent magnet is an alloy of aluminium, nickel, and cobalt, known as *alnico*.

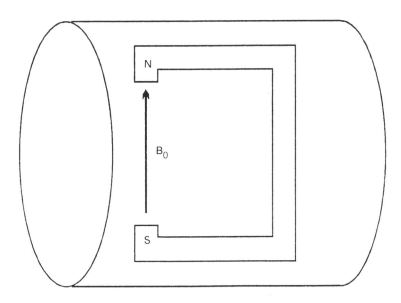

Fig. 9.5 The field of a permanent magnet.

The main advantage of permanent magnets is that they require no power supply and are therefore low in operating costs. In addition, the magnetic field created by a permanent magnet has lines of flux running vertically from the south to the north pole (bottom to the top) of the magnet, keeping the magnetic field virtually confined within the boundaries of the scan room (Fig. 9.5). Also such systems can be designed with open configurations. Despite the low field strengths and associated lower SNR, open systems have become popular for claustrophobic and obese patients, kinematic musculoskeletal studies and interventional procedures, all of which are difficult in a closed solenoid configuration.

Electromagnets

The laws of electromagnetism state that moving electrical charges induce magnetic fields around themselves. Therefore, if a current (or a moving charge) is passed through a long straight wire, a magnetic field is created around that wire (Fig. 9.6). The strength of the resultant magnetic field is proportional to the amount of current moving through the wire. The magnetic field strength created by introducing current through a wire is calculated by the following equation

$$B_0 = k\,I$$

where I is the current, k is the proportionality constant (quantity of charge on each body), and B_0 is the magnetic field strength.

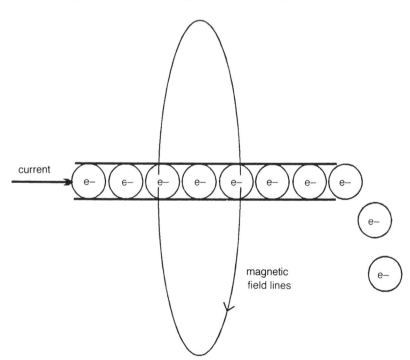

Fig. 9.6 Flow of electrons along a wire and the induced magnetic field.

Therefore the current passing along the wire is proportional to the magnetic field induced around it. The direction of the magnetic field induced can be expressed by the right hand thumb rule. This rule states that if the fingers of the right hand are curled around a wire and the thumb points in the direction of the current, the fingers point in the direction of the magnetic field.

If current is passed through two parallel straight wires in opposing directions, the two magnetic fields tend to cancel out each other in the region between the two wires. Conversely, if the current passing along the parallel wires is flowing in the same direction, contributions to the resultant magnetic field are additive. This property is exploited for the generation of large magnetic fields.

Solenoid electromagnets

Instead of using several parallel wires, one wire can be wrapped around to form many loops like a spring. The loops of wire form a coil and act as though they are parallel straight wires. The strength of the resultant magnetic field of the coil is expressed by the equation

$$B_0 = 2\pi \, kNI/R$$

where N is the number of closely spaced loops, and R is the radius of the loops.

This is called a *solenoidal electromagnet* and as the loops of wire appear to be evenly spaced, the magnetic field in this solenoidal magnet is considerably uniform that it generates similar field strengths from one end to the other.

A factor that governs the efficiency of the passage of current is the inherent resistance of the coil. The degree of resistance along a wire is determined by *Ohm's law*. Ohm's law states

$$V = IR$$

where V is equal to the applied voltage (which for our purposes is constant), I is the current, and R is the resistance within the wire.

Therefore, the solenoidal electromagnet is often said to be a *resistive magnet*.

Resistive magnets

The magnetic field strength in a resistive magnet is dependent upon the current which passes through its coils of wire. The direction of the main magnetic field in a resistive magnet follows the right-hand thumb rule, and produces lines of flux running horizontally from the head to the foot of the magnet (Fig. 9.7). As a resistive system primarily consists of loops carrying current, it is lighter in weight than the permanent magnet and although its capital costs are low, the operational costs of the resistive magnet are quite high due to the large quantities of power required to maintain the magnetic field. Therefore the maximum field strength in a system of this type is less than 0.3 T due to its excessive power requirements. The resistive system is relatively safe as the field can be turned off instantly with the flick of a switch. However, this type of magnet does create significant stray magnetic fields. (Stray magnetic fields and magnetic field shielding are discussed later in this chapter.)

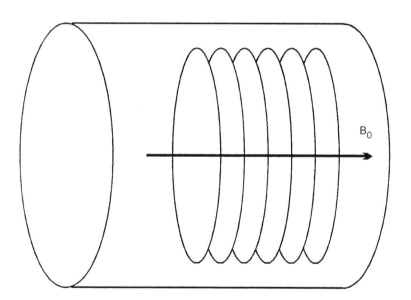

Fig. 9.7 The field of a solenoidal magnet.

Super conducting electromagnets

As resistance decreases, the current dissipation also decreases. Therefore if the resistance is reduced, the energy required to maintain the magnetic field is decreased. Resistance is dependent upon the material of which the loops of wire are made, the length of the wire in the loop, and the cross-sectional area of the wire itself. In addition, resistance is dependent on the temperature of the wires, which can be controlled so that resistance is minimised. In particular, some materials called superconductors exhibit zero resistance below a certain very low temperature. This is called the critical temperature. These wires are used to make the wires of superconducting magnets. A widely used material is an alloy of niobium and titanium which becomes superconductive below approximately 4 K (Kelvin).

Initially, current is passed through the loops of wire to create the magnetic field or bring the field up to strength (ramping). Then the wires are super cooled with substances known as *cryogens* (usually liquid helium (He) to eliminate resistance. This is called a *cryogen bath* which actually surrounds the coils of wire and is housed in the system between insulated vacuums.

When used to produce MR images, the super conducting magnet produces relatively high magnetic field strengths with low power requirements (after the magnetic field has been ramped up). With resistance virtually eliminated, there is no longer a mechanism to dissipate current, therefore no additional power input is required to maintain the high magnetic field strength. Although the super conducting magnet has a relatively low operating cost, a system of this type is expensive to buy. However, the super conducting system offers extremely high field strengths of 0.5 to 4 T for clinical imaging, and anything up to 9 T for spectroscopic and high resolution studies. The direction of the main magnetic field runs horizontally like that of the resistive system, from the head to the feet of the patient.

- Permanent magnets:
        Remain magnetised permanently
        Flux lines run vertically
        Require no power supply
        Low operational costs
        Small fringe fields
        Heavy
        Low field strengths (SNR lower/usually longer scan times)
- Resistive magnets:
        Field can be switched off immediately
        Flux lines horizontal
        High operational cost as power supply required
        Large fringe fields
        Low field strengths (SNR lower/usually longer scan times)
- Super conducting magnets:
        Flux lines horizontal
        Lower power requirements (cheap to run)
        Expensive to buy
        Large fringe fields
        High field strength (higher SNR/usually shorter scan times)

Fringe fields

The static magnetic field has no respect for the confines of conventional walls, floors or ceilings. The stray magnetic field outside the bore of the magnet is known as the *fringe field*. All magnets have a fringe field to some extent. The field associated with a permanent magnet is relatively low but in solenoid electromagnets, the fringe field is significant. These fringe fields must therefore be taken into account when siting a magnet, so that they do not extend into areas where potentially contraindicated patients, monitoring devices and other mechanical and magnetically activated devices are present.

Shielding

Fringe fields can be compensated for by the use of magnetic field shielding. MR systems can be shielded by two processes which are:

(1) passive shielding,
(2) active shielding.

Passive shielding can be accomplished by lining the walls of the MR scan room with steel. These techniques are low in cost and offer effective confinement of the magnetic field. The more expensive alternative is active shielding which uses additional solenoid magnets outside the cryogen bath that restrict the magnetic field lines to an acceptable location. Some manufacturers offer actively shielded magnets which reduce the stray fields to an area as small as one quarter of a tennis court. This facilitates the siting of systems in very small spaces such as trucks. Unshielded magnets require a large building so that fringe fields do not extend beyond its walls.

Shim coils

Due to design limitations it is almost impossible to create an electromagnet which produces a perfectly homogeneous magnetic field (Fig. 9.8). To correct for these inhomogeneities, either a piece of metal or other loops of current carrying wire are placed around the bore. This process is called *shimming* and the extra loop of wire is called a *shim coil*. When the magnet is shimmed with metal it is termed passive shimming; when shimming is performed with loops of current carrying wire it is known as active shimming. Both passive and active shimming produce magnetic field evenness or homogeneity. For imaging purposes, homogeneity of the order of 10 ppm is required. Spectroscopic procedures require a more homogeneous environment of 1 ppm.

The shim system requires a power supply which is separate from the other power supplies within the system. This is important because a fault in the shim power supply compromises image quality.

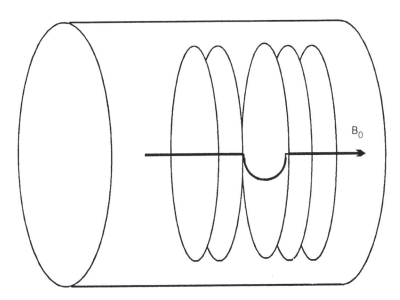

Fig. 9.8 Inhomogeneity of the main magnetic field.

Gradient coils

As previously described, the magnetic field strength is proportional to the amount of current passed through the loop of wire, the number of loops in the wire, the size of the loops, and how closely the loops are spaced. If the loops are spaced closely at one end of the solenoid and gradually become farther apart at the other end, the resultant magnetic field becomes stronger at one end than the other. This is called a *magnetic field gradient*. Gradient coils provide a linear gradation or slope of the magnetic field strength from one end of the solenoid to the other (Fig. 9.9). The gradients are applied by passing current through the gradient coil in a certain direction. This either increases or decreases the magnetic field strength on either side of the isocentre. The amplitude of the gradient slope is determined by the magnitude of the current passing through the coil.

By varying the magnetic field strength, gradients provide position-dependent variation of signal frequency and are therefore used for slice selection, frequency encoding, phase encoding, rewinding and spoiling. Gradient coils are powered by gradient amplifiers. Faults in the gradient coils or gradient amplifiers can result in geometric distortions in the MR image.

Gradient strength can be expressed in units of G/cm or mT/m where

$$1 \text{ G/cm} = 10 \text{ mT/m}$$

This means that the magnetic field changes by 1 gauss over each centimetre or 10 milli tesla over each metre. Stronger gradients (15 or 20 mT/m) permit high speed or high resolution imaging (see Chapter 12).

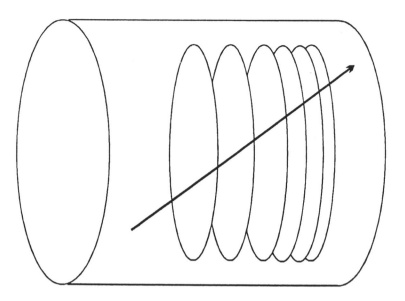

Fig. 9.9 A gradient coil.

Radio-frequency coils

The energy required to produce resonance of nuclear spins is expressed as a frequency and can be calculated by the Larmor equation. At field strengths used in MRI, energy within the radio frequency (RF) band of the electromagnetic spectrum is necessary to perturb or excite the spins. As shown by the Larmor equation, the magnetic field strength is proportional to the radio frequency, the energy of which is significantly lower than that of X-rays. In order to produce an image, RF must first be transmitted at the resonant frequency of hydrogen so that resonance can occur. The transverse component of magnetisation created by resonance must then be detected by a receiver coil.

RF transmitters

Energy is transmitted at the resonant frequency of hydrogen in the form of a short intense burst of radio frequency known as a radio-frequency pulse. This is achieved by a radio-transmitter which sends frequency with enough energy to force phase coherence and flip some of the spins from a low to a high energy state. This RF pulse transfers the NMV from a position parallel to B_0, to an orientation at right angles to B_0. Such a pulse is therefore called a 90° RF pulse.

The 90° RF pulse is created by an oscillating secondary magnetic field (B_1) formed as a result of passing current through a loop of wire called a RF transmitter coil (Fig. 9.10). To accomplish excitation, the secondary B_1 field must be situated at right angles to the main magnetic field B_0. The main magnetic field of a permanent magnet is usually vertical, whereas a solenoidal type of magnet has horizontal flux lines. Therefore the

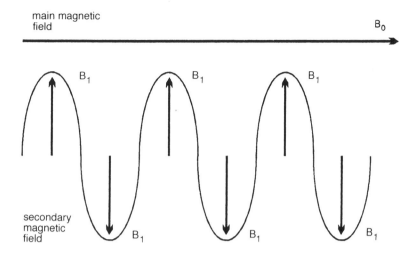

Fig. 9.10 Static versus secondary magnetic field.

secondary field of the RF coil should occur in the horizontal axis in permanent magnets, and in the transverse or vertical axes in solenoidal magnets. As shown by the laws of electromagnetism, this field is created perpendicular to the transmitter coils themselves. In practice when using solenoidal electromagnets, for example, the RF transmitter coil should be oriented above, below, or at the sides of the patient. For this reason, RF transmitter coils used in electromagnets are usually cylindrical (Fig. 9.11). The main RF transmitter coils in most systems are:

(1) a body coil usually located within the bore of the magnet itself,
(2) a head coil which is coupled to a receiver coil.

The body coil is the main RF transmitter and transmits RF for most examinations that are acquired without a transmit receive coil. Typical transmit receive coils are head, extremity and some breast coils.

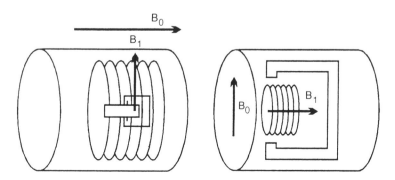

Fig. 9.11 Transmitter coil field of permanent and electromagnets.

Receiver coils

As previously discussed, passing current through a wire produces a magnetic field. Conversely, if a loop of wire is exposed to an oscillating field, a current is induced in the loop. This induced current and the resulting voltage constitute the MR signal. Receiver coils must be placed properly in order to adequately detect the MR signal.

RF coil types

The configuration of the RF transmitter and receiver probes or coils directly affects the quality of the MR signal. There are several types of coil currently used in MR imaging. These are:

(1) the volume coil or bird-cage coil,
(2) the surface coil,
(3) phased array coil,
(4) the solenoidal coil,
(5) the Helmholtz pair.

The three most common coils in use are now discussed.

Volume coils

A volume coil can both transmit RF and receive the MR signal and is often called a transceiver. It encompasses the entire anatomy and can be used for either head, extremity or total body imaging. Head and body coils of a type known as the bird-cage configuration are used to image relatively large areas and yield uniform SNR over the entire imaging volume. However, even though volume coils are responsible for uniform excitation over a large area, because of their large size they generally produce images with lower SNR than other types of coils.

The signal quality produced by volume coils has been significantly increased by the advent of a process known as *quadrature excitation and detection*. This enables signal to be transmitted and received by two pairs of coils. In most cases quadrature coils are used to transmit RF as well as to receive the MR signal.

Surface coils

Coils of this type are used to improve the SNR when imaging structures near the surface of the patient (such as the lumbar spine). Generally, the nearer the coil is situated to the structure under examination, the greater the SNR. This is because the coil is closer to the signal-emitting anatomy, and only noise in the vicinity of the coil is received rather than the entire body. Surface coils are usually small and especially shaped so that they can be easily placed near the anatomy to be imaged with little or no discomfort to the patient. However, signal (and noise) is received only from the sensitive volume of the coil which corresponds to the area located around the coil. The size of this area extends to the circumference of the coil and at a depth into the patient equal to the radius of the coil. There is therefore a fall off of signal as the distance from the coil is increased in any direction. However, with the recent advent of intra-cavity coils (such as rectal coils), surface or local coils as they are often now called, can be used to receive signal deep within the patient. As the SNR is enhanced when using local coils, greater spatial resolution of small structures can often be achieved. When using local coils, the body coil is used to transmit RF and the local coil is used to receive the MR signal.

- Large coil:
  - Large area of uniform signal reception
  - Increased likelihood of aliasing with small FOV
  - Positioning of patient not too critical
  - Lower SNR and resolution
  - Used in examinations of torso where signal coverage is necessary (chest, abdomen)
- Small coil:
  - Small area of signal reception
  - Less likely to produce aliasing artefact
  - Positioning of coil and patient critical
  - High SNR and resolution
  - Used in examinations of small body parts (wrist, spine, knee)

Phased array coils

Phased array coils are now widely used. These consist of multiple coils and receivers whose individual signals are combined to create one image with improved SNR and increased coverage. Therefore the advantages of small surface coils (increased SNR and resolution), can be combined with a large FOV for increased anatomy coverage. Usually up to four coils and receivers are grouped together to increase either longitudinal coverage (for spine imaging), or to improve uniformity across a whole volume (pelvic imaging). During data acquisition, each individual coil receives signal from its own small usable FOV. The signal output from each coil is separately received and processed but then combined to form one single larger FOV. As each coil has its own receiver the amount of noise received is limited to its small FOV, and all the data can be acquired in a single sequence rather than four individual ones. There are several types of phased array coils now available. These include:

(1) spine phased array,
(2) pelvic phased array,

(3) breast coil phased array,
(4) tempero-mandibular joint phased array.

Coil safety

There are a few basic rules to ensure the safe operation of RF coils. Coils are connected to the system by cables which must consist of a conductive material so that the RF power can be delivered to the coil and the signal can be sent to the image processor. They therefore have the capacity to transmit heat which occurs during normal operation. However under certain circumstances, this heat may burn the patient or the insulating material of the cable. To prevent such an occurrence, always ensure that the cables are not looped and do not touch the patient or the bore of the magnet. Coil cables should be inspected regularly and should not under any circumstances be used if the insulation is damaged. To receive optimum signal from the patient, the coils must be correctly tuned. Each manufacturer has his own method of achieving this.

Now that the individual components of the magnet system have been discussed, the larger hardware elements are now described.

The pulse control unit

Gradient coils are switched on and off very rapidly and at precise times during the pulse sequence. They not only spatially localise signal along the three axes of the magnet, but are also used to rewind or spoil transverse magnetisation and to rephase magnetisation. The same three gradients perform all these tasks and accurate pulsing of the gradient coils is essential. *Gradient amplifiers* supply the power to the gradient coils and a *pulse control unit* co-ordinates the functions of the gradient amplifiers and the coils so that they can be switched on and off at the appropriate times.

The pulse control unit is also responsible for co-ordinating the transmission and amplification of the RF. RF at the resonant frequency is transmitted by the RF transceiver to the RF amplifier and then through an RF monitor which ensures that safe levels of RF are delivered to the patient.

The received RF signal from the coil is amplified and then passes to the array processor for Fast Fourier Transform. This data is then transmitted to the image processor so that each pixel can be allocated a grey scale colour in the image.

Patient transportation system

All systems use a hydraulically or mechanically driven couch to lift the patient up to the level of the bore and to slide them into the magnet. This is usually achieved by pedals or buttons that move the couch up or down, and in or out of the bore. The table should be comfortable for the patient and allow for the attachment of coils and immobilisation devices. There should also be a mechanism for evacuating the patient rapidly from the bore in an emergency. Some systems enable the couch to be undocked from the magnet, so that patients can be transported out of the room in an emergency without moving them on to another trolley first. All couches must of course, be magnetically safe and contain no metal parts.

Operator interface

MRI computer systems vary with manufacturer. Most however consist of:

- a minicomputer with expansion capabilities,
- an array processor for Fourier transformation,
- an image processor that takes data from the array processor to form an image,
- hard disc drives for storage of raw data and pulse sequence parameters,
- a power distribution mechanism to distribute and filter the alternating and direct current.

The operator's link to the system exists in the form of a boot terminal usually in the vicinity of the minicomputer. System initialisation and software modifications can be accessed with the use of this terminal. However, scanning and viewing capabilities are accessed at an operator's console, usually located directly outside of the scan room.

In addition to data acquisition and viewing the recently acquired images, the operator console provides access to a whole host of image manipulation techniques. These techniques include:

(1) viewing several images at the same time,
(2) viewing images in a cine loop,
(3) reformatting 3D volume images.

MR images are permanently stored from the image console on to single emulsion film similar to that used in computed tomography. However, filming MR images can be somewhat tricky in that the brightness and contrast settings vary with each image. These brightness and contrast settings are referred to as *window and level settings*. Images with high intrinsic signal may require different window and level settings so that important anatomic and pathologic findings may be visualised adequately on the MR image.

For permanent storage of MR image data, data may be archived on to either *magnetic tape*, *dat tape* or *optical disk*. This archive function can also be accessed through the operator's console. Images are stored so that cases can be retrieved for further manipulation and imaging in the future. They may also be used for comparison when repeat examinations are performed on the same patient.

Now that each component of the equipment has been described, it is appropriate to discuss the safe operation of this equipment. This is the subject of the next chapter.

Questions

1. Name the system components responsible for the production of the B_1 field:
   (a) main magnet coils
   (b) gradient coils
   (c) RF coils
   (d) shim coils.

2. The process that changes the RF signal from a FID to a spectrum is called:
   (a) Fourier transform
   (b) Larmor equation
   (c) Faraday's laws of induction
   (d) Ohm's law.

3. In solenoid electromagnets, the strength of the magnetic field is dependent upon:
   (a) the distance between the current carrying loops of wire
   (b) the number of closely spaced loops
   (c) the amount of current passed through a wire
   (d) all of the above.

4. Shim coils provide a means for:
   (a) magnetic field homogeneity
   (b) position dependent variation of field strength and signal frequency
   (c) a static magnetic field
   (d) an oscillating magnetic field.

5. Complete the sentence. ... provide optimal coverage and SNR for spine imaging.
   (a) Surface coils
   (b) Head coils
   (c) Phased array coils
   (d) Volume coils.

6. Homogeneity is generally expressed in units of:
   (a) G/cm
   (b) mT/m
   (c) W/kg
   (d) ppm.

7. Permanent, open systems are being designed for:
   (a) claustrophobics
   (b) interventional procedures
   (c) kinematic studies
   (d) all of the above.

Chapter 10   MRI Safety

Introduction

As yet, virtually no long term adverse biological effects of extended exposure to MRI have been described. However, on examination of the separate components of the magnetic resonance imaging process, several inconsequential and reversible effects of magnetic, gradient and radio frequency fields can be observed. Much of the research into MR safety has been carried out in the US and it is from there that most of the literature on safety originates. In February 1982, the Food and Drug Administration (FDA) issued guidelines to Hospital's Investigational Review Boards (IRBs) in 'Guidelines for Evaluating Electromagnetic Exposure Risks for Trials of Clinical NMR'. The 1988 version of this is the latest and most pertinent data for safety (see Federal Register 1988). This was later followed up with an evaluation of potential risks and hazards. In order to discuss the long-term biological effects of MRI, all the components of the imaging process must be considered. Those elements include

(1) the main magnetic field (also known as the static magnetic field),
(2) time varying magnetic fields (magnetic field gradients and RF fields),
(3) radio frequency fields (RF coils).

It should be noted that all patients and personnel must be screened before entering the scan room. The International Society for Magnetic Resonance in Medicine (ISMRM) has issued a screening form that should be used as a guideline for screening all persons who enter the MR suite.

The main magnetic field

The main magnetic field is responsible for the alignment of nuclei. In solenoid electromagnets the field is usually horizontal, whereas in

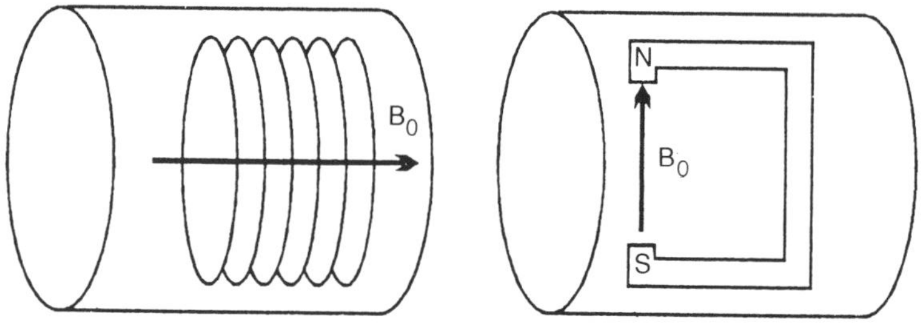

Fig. 10.1 The main magnetic field of an electromagnet and a permanent magnet.

permanent magnets the field is generally vertical (Fig. 10.1). This is a static or unchanging field. The FDA limit for static magnetic field strength is 2 T for clinical imaging. Higher field strengths are permitted for research.

Biological effects of the static magnetic field

The primary concern with the static magnetic field is the possibility of potential biological effects. In nature, the magnetic field associated with the earth does have significant effect on lower life forms. The orientation of magneto-static bacteria and the migratory patterns of birds, are influenced by the 0.6 G magnetic field which surrounds the earth. In MR, small electrical potentials have been observed in large blood vessels which flow perpendicular to the static magnetic field. However even at 10 T, no adverse effects have been noted on the ECGs of squirrel monkeys. The majority of studies show no effects on cell growth and morphology at field strengths below 2 T. Data accumulated by the National Institute for Occupational Safety, the World Health Organization, and the US State Department, show no evidence of leukaemia or other carcinogenesis. However, the *New England Journal of Medicine* reported an increase in leukaemia in men exposed to electrical and magnetic fields in Washington State, from 1950 to 1979, in these cases the electromagnetic fields were produced by alternating currents which resulted in changing magnetic fields. Although similar effects were detected in New York in 1987, no evidence of adverse effects have been noted in persons working with linear accelerators who are exposed to static magnetic fields. The few reports of potential carcinogenesis seem controversial, in that many of the study methods have been criticised.

Fringe fields

The secondary concern of the effects of the main magnetic field is the hazards associated with the siting of MR systems. The static magnetic field has no respect for the confines of conventional walls, floors or ceilings. This stray magnetic field outside the bore of the magnet, is known as the fringe field (Fig. 10.2).

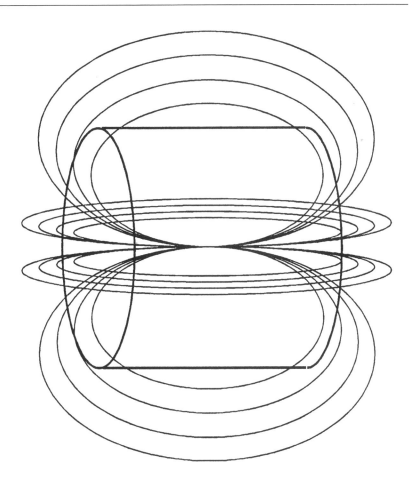

Fig. 10.2   The fringe field.

Most magnetic resonance imagers are shielded to confine the fringe field to an acceptable location, either within the scan room or (in the case of mobile MR systems), within the confines of the truck. However, the fringe field must always be taken into consideration when siting new systems. The field strength above and below the system should also be considered when siting, to prevent the untimely demise of a painter with a pacemaker who inadvertently climbs a ladder to paint the ceiling! It is therefore recommended that the general public (those persons who have not been properly screened for the effects of magnetic fields) remain out of the field strength below 5 G. For this reason many imaging facilities are situated so that public areas are below this strength, and areas above are either inaccessible or clearly marked.

Static fields below 2.0 T

Although no biological effects have been observed in human subjects at field strengths below 2 T, reversible effects have been noted on ECGs at these field strengths. An increase in the amplitude of the T-wave can be noted on an ECG due to the magnetohydrodynamic effect. This is produced when a conductive fluid, such as blood, moves across a magnetic field. It is proportional to the strength of the magnetic field. This effect is considered reversible as the ECG tracing returns to normal when the patient is removed from the field. The magnetic haemodynamic effect can present problems when cardiac gating in high field systems. It results in the system triggering from the T-wave rather than the R-wave, and so image quality suffers as a result of insufficient cardiac gating. However despite this effect, no serious cardiovascular effects have been observed in patients undergoing MR.

Static fields above 2.0 T

Some reversible biological effects have been observed on human subjects exposed to 2.0 T and above. These effects include fatigue, headaches, hypotension and accounts of irritability. Another potential problem at these higher field strengths is the effect of magnetic interaction energy and cell orientation. Certain molecules (such as DNA) and cellular sub-units (such as sickled red cells), have magnetic properties that vary with direction. This effect is biologically important at a field strength of 2.0 T, because of the twisting force or torque that is exerted on these molecules.

Pregnant patients

As yet, there are no known biological effects of MRI on fetuses. However, there are a number of mechanisms that could potentially cause adverse effects as a result of the interaction of electromagnetic fields with developing fetuses. Cells undergoing division, which occurs during the first trimester of pregnancy are more susceptible to these effects.

The FDA requires labelling of MR systems to indicate the safety of MR when used to image the fetus and infant. The current recommendation by the FDA states 'If the information to be gained by MR would have required more invasive testing, MRI is acceptable'. In the light of the high risk potential for pregnant patients in general, many facilities prefer to delay any examination of pregnant patients until the first trimester and then have a written consent form signed before the examination, by the patient. In addition, the American College of Gynaecology and Obstetrics, recommends that pregnant patients should be reviewed on a case by case basis. The Society of Magnetic Resonance Imaging Safety committee suggests that 'Pregnant patients or those who suspect they are pregnant, should be identified before undergoing MRI in order to assesss the relative risks versus the benefits of the examination.'

In Great Britain, The National Radiological Protection Board (NRPB) guidelines specify that '. . . it might be prudent to exclude pregnant women during the first three months of pregnancy'. However it should be noted, that numerous fetuses have undergone MRI since 1983 without any abnormalities at birth, or after four years of childhood development. Gadolinium enhancement is at present best avoided when examining a pregnant patient.

Pregnant employees

MR facilities have established individual guidelines for pregnant employees in the magnetic resonance environment. The safety committee of the ISMRM determined that pregnant employees can safely enter the scan room, but should leave while the RF and gradient fields are employed. Some facilities however, recommend that the employee stay out of the magnetic field entirely during the first trimester of pregnancy.

A recent survey shows no increased incidence of spontaneous abortions among MR radiographers and nurses, (it should be noted that the natural incidence of spontaneous abortions is roughly 30%). Following this survey, the unit that carried out the study changed their in-house policy from one in which radiographers were kept out of the magnetic field during pregnancy, to a policy which allows pregnant radiographers and technologists to set up the patient, but not to remain during image acquisition. It has been suggested that informed workers make their own decision. In the US, this recommendation was influenced by a legal decision concerning the rights of pregnant workers in hazardous environments. It seems therefore, that MR is too new to make an informed decision on magnetic safety for pregnant radiographers. Each person must make their own decision to either stay in the unit or if possible, to rotate back into a nearby radiology department. However, to leave an environment which is probably safe, into one which is known to be hazardous, may be inadvisable!

Projectiles

Ferromagnetic metal objects can become airborne as projectiles in the presence of a strong static magnetic field. Small objects, such as paper clips and hair pins, have a terminal velocity of 40 mph when pulled into a 1.5 T magnet, and therefore pose a serious risk to the patient and anyone else present in the scan room. The force with which projectiles are pulled toward a magnetic field is proportional to the mass of the object and the distance from the magnet. Even surgical tools such as haemostats, scissors and clamps, although made of a material known as 'surgical stainless steel', are strongly attracted to the main magnetic field. Oxygen tanks are also highly magnetic and should never be brought into the scan room. However there are non-ferrous oxygen tanks available which are safe. Sand bags must also be inspected since some are filled, not with sand, but with steel shot which is highly magnetic.

It is recommended that all objects are tested with a hand-held bar magnet before entering the MR scan room. In addition, it is advised that all nursing, housekeeping, fire department, emergency and MR personnel are educated about the potential risks and hazards of the static magnetic field. Signs should be attached at all entrances to the magnetic field (including the fringe field), to deter entry into the scan room with ferromagnetic objects. Metal detectors are available, but can in some cases offer a false sense of security. For this reason, most imaging facilities keep the general public well behind the 5 G line.

Medical emergencies

As in any medical facility, the MR suite should be equipped with emergency medical supplies on a crash cart. Many of these supplies can be incredibly dangerous in an MR environment. For this reason, in any critical situation, it is recommended that the patient is rapidly removed from the magnetic field before resuscitation begins.

Implants and prostheses

Metallic implants pose serious effects which include torque, heating and artefacts on MR images. Therefore before imaging patients with MR, any surgical procedure that the patient has undergone prior to the MR examination must be identified. For a complete list of MR compatible implants and prosthesis refer to *Magnetic Resonance Bioeffects, Safety and Patient Management* by Shellock and Kanal (1996).

Torque and heating

Some metallic implants have shown considerable torque when placed in the presence of a magnetic field. The force or torque exerted on small and large metallic implants can cause serious effects, as unanchored implants can potentially move unpredictably within the body. The type of metal used in such implants, is one factor which determines the force exerted on them in magnetic fields. While non-ferrous metallic implants may show little or no deflection to the field, they could cause significant heating due to their inability to dissipate the heat caused by radio-frequency absorption.

However, heating experiments have not shown excessive temperature increases in implants.

Artefacts from metallic implants

Although artefacts cannot be considered as a biological effect of the MR process, misinterpretation of MR images can yield devastating consequences. It should be noted that the type of metal, as well as size of the metallic implant, and the pulse sequence used determines the size of the artefact on the MR image. Therefore, if a metal artefact is seen and no metal is present within the patient, this could indicate the presence of blood products suggestive of a haemorrhagic lesion.

Intra-cranial vascular clips

Some intra-cranial aneurysm clips are absolute contraindications in MR imaging. Clip motion may damage the vessel, resulting in haemorrhage, ischaemia or death. Intra-cranial clips made of a material known as titanium have been used, and have proved safe for MR. Unfortunately there have been several cases where a clip was either 'MR compatible' or thought to be and the clip moved during an MR scan resulting in death. It is therefore recommended by the ISMRM that imaging of patients with aneurysm clips is not performed unless the clip has been tested for magnetic safety prior to insertion.

Intra-vascular coils, filters and stents

Fifteen intra-vascular devices have been tested and five of these proved to be ferromagnetic. Although they have shown deflection in the magnetic field, these devices usually become imbedded in the vessel wall after several weeks, and are unlikely to become dislodged. Therefore it is considered safe to perform MR imaging on most patients with intra-vascular devices, provided a reasonable period of time has elapsed after implantation.

Extra-cranial vascular clips

Five carotid artery vascular clamps have been tested and each showed deflection in the magnetic field. However, the deflection was mild when compared with the pulsatile vascular motion within the carotids. Extra-cranial clips tend to be surrounded by fibrous tissue or scar after surgery. It is recommended that MR is delayed until 4–6 weeks after surgery but all studies should be evaluated on a case-by-case basis. Only the Poppen–Blaylock carotid artery clamp is believed to be contraindicated for MR, due to its large attractive response to the magnetic field.

Vascular access ports

Only two of the thirty three implanted vascular access ports recently tested showed measurable deflection in the magnetic field. These deflections are thought to be insignificant to the applications of such ports. Therefore, it is probably safe to image patients with implanted vascular access ports.

Heart valves

Twenty five of the twenty nine heart valve prostheses have been evaluated for magnetic susceptibility, and these showed negligible deflection to the magnetic field. The deflection is minimal compared with normal pulsatile cardiac motion. Therefore, although patients with most valvular implants are considered safe for MR, careful screening for valve type is advised because there are valves whose integrity could be compromised.

Dental devices and materials

Sixteen dental implants have been tested and twelve of these have shown measurable deflection to the magnetic field, however most are thought to be safe for MR imaging. Although most devices are not significantly affected by the magnetic field, susceptibility artefacts can adversely affect image quality in MR especially in gradient echo imaging. It should be noted that some dental devices are magnetically activated, and therefore can pose potential risks for MR imaging.

Penile implants

Only one of the nine penile implants recently tested showed measurable deflection to the magnetic field. This, the Dacomed Omniphase is unlikely to cause severe damage to the patient, but may become uncomfortable and so an alternative imaging procedure may be considered.

Otologic implants

All three cochlear implants recently tested were attracted to the magnetic field and were magnetically or electronically activated. They are therefore definitely contraindicated for MRI. Some patients with otologic implants have been issued a card warning them to avoid MR imaging.

Ocular implants

Of twelve ocular implants tested, two were deflected by a 1.5 T static magnetic field. The Fatio eyelid spring could cause discomfort and the retinal tack could injure the eye since it is made from a ferromagnetic form of stainless steel.

Intra-ocular ferrous foreign bodies

Intra-ocular ferrous foreign bodies are a cause of major concern in MR safety. It is not uncommon for patients who have worked with sheet metal to have metal fragments or slivers located in and around the eye. Since the magnetic field exerts a force on ferromagnetic objects, a metal fragment in the eye could move or be displaced and cause injury to the eye or surrounding tissue. Small intra-ocular fragments could be missed on a standard radiograph. However, a recent study demonstrated that metal fragments as small as $0.1 \times 0.1 \times 0.1$ mm can be detected on standard radiographs. In addition, metal fragments from $0.1 \times 0.1 \times 0.1$ mm to $0.3 \times 0.1 \times 0.1$ mm were examined in the eyes of laboratory animals in a 2.0 T magnet. Only the $0.3 \times 0.1 \times 0.1$ mm fragments moved, but they did not cause any discernible clinical damage. Therefore, although computed tomography is more accurate in detecting the presence of small foreign bodies, plain film radiography should be adequate in screening for intra-ocular ferrous foreign bodies that have sufficient size to cause ocular damage.

The ISMRM screening form asks the patient 'Have you ever been hit in the eye by metal?' This is worded in such a way to imply that even if they once had metal in their eye and thought it had been removed they should still be screened with plain X-rays. It is also recommended that two views are obtained for evaluation of the orbits. Such views include a 20° posterior–anterior (Water's view) and a lateral or two Water's views with the eyes looking up and down.

Bullets, pellets and shrapnel

Although the majority of ammunition has proved to be non-ferrous, ammunition made in some countries or produced by the military, has shown traces of ferromagnetic alloys. Therefore, it is advisable to take extreme caution in imaging patient with bullets or shrapnel, and to be aware of the location of such metal within the body.

Orthopaedic implants, materials and devices

Each of fifteen orthopaedic implants recently tested showed no deflection within the main magnetic field. However a large metallic implant such as a hip prosthesis, can become heated by currents induced in the metal by the magnetic and radio frequency fields. It appears however, that such heating is relatively low. The majority of orthopaedic implants have been imaged with MR without incident.

Surgical clips and pins

Abdominal surgical clips are generally safe for MR because they become anchored by fibrous tissue but produce artefacts in proportion to their size and can distort the image. It is recommended that, if possible, the MR procedure is delayed until 4–6 weeks post-operative. As always, patients should be evaluated on a case-by-case basis.

Halo vests and other similar externally applied devices

Halo vests pose several risk factors which include deflection and subsequent dislodging of the halo, heating due to RF absorption, electrical current induction within the halo rings, electrical arcing and severe artefactual consequences which could render the imaging acquisition useless. Non-ferrous and non-conductive halo vests which are MR compatible are commercially available. Therefore, in the light of the potential risks and hazards associated with halo vests, it is advisable to identify the halo vest before proceeding with MR imaging.

Electrically, magnetically or mechanically activated or electrically conductive implanted devices

Certain implanted devices are contraindicated for MR imaging because they are either magnetically, electrically or mechanically activated. These implants include:

(1) cardiac pacemakers (pacemakers will be discussed later in more detail),
(2) cochlear implants,
(3) tissue expanders,
(4) ocular prostheses,
(5) dental implants,
(6) neurostimulators,
(7) bone growth stimulators,
(8) implantable cardiac defibrillators,
(9) implantable drug infusion pumps.

The function of such implants is impaired by the magnetic field, therefore patients with such devices should not be examined with MR. Also, devices which depend on magnetisation to affix themselves to the patient (such as magnetic sphincters, magnetic stoma plugs and magnetic prosthetic devices), could be demagnetised and may be contraindicated for MR.

Pacemakers

Cardiac pacemakers are an absolute contraindication for MRI. Even field strengths as low as 5 G may be sufficient to cause deflection, programming changes, and closure of the reed switch which converts a pacemaker to an asynchronous mode. In addition, patients who have had their pacemaker removed may have pacer wires left within the body which could act as an antenna, and (by induced currents), cause cardiac fibrillation. Warning signs should be posted at the 5 G line to prevent the exposure of anyone with a pacemaker or other electronic implants.

Gradient magnetic fields

All MR imaging systems are equipped with a set of resistive wire windings known as gradient coils. Gradients provide position-dependent variation in magnetic field strength and are pulsed on and off during and between RF excitation pulses. The purpose of these gradients is spatially to encode information contained in the emitted RF signal. However, in doing so, they create a time-varying magnetic field (TVMF).

Time-varying magnetic fields

There have been a large number of studies performed on the biological effects from TVMF, since they exist around power transformers and high voltage lines. The health consequences are not related to the strength of the gradient field, but rather to changes in the magnetic field that cause induced currents. In MR, there is concern with nerves, blood vessels and muscles that act as conductors in the body. Faraday's law of induction states that changing magnetic fields induce electrical currents in any conducting medium. Induced currents are proportional to the material's conductivity and the rate of change of the magnetic field. In MR, this effect is determined by factors such as pulse duration, wave shape, repetition pattern, and the distribution of the current in the body. The induced current is greater in peripheral tissues since the amplitude of the gradient is higher away from magnetic isocentre.

Biological effects which vary with current amplitude, range from reversible alterations in vision, to irreversible effects of cardiac fibrillation, alterations in the biochemistry of cells and fracture union. Effects occasionally experienced during MRI examinations using echo planar techniques include mild cutaneous sensations and involuntary muscle contractions. Visual effects may occur when retinal phosphenes are stimulated by induction from TVMF. This results in light flashes or 'stars in one's eyes'. The FDA limit for TVMF is expressed in the same units as Faraday's laws of induction. In the Faraday equation:

$$dB/dT = dV$$

where dB is the change in magnetic field (caused by switching gradients), dT is the change in time and dV is the change in voltage.

The FDA limit for gradient field is 6 T/s for all gradients. In this case, therefore, dB is 6 T and dT is 1 s. In addition, the FDA limits axial gradient fields to 20 T/s and gradient rise times to 120 ms. EPI sequences pose the greatest concern for TVMF effects as strong gradients are switched rapidly during image acquisition.

Acoustic noise

As current is passed through the gradient coils during image acquisition, a significant amount of acoustic noise is created. Although noise levels on most commercial systems, is considered to be within recommended safety guidelines, it can cause some reversible and irreversible effects. These effects include communication interference, patient annoyance, transient hearing loss and in patients who are susceptible to hearing impairment, permanent hearing loss. Ear plugs are an acceptable and inexpensive way of preventing hearing loss and should be used regularly. In fact it is recommended that all patients are provided with ear plugs or head phones. A more expensive alternative is 'anti-noise' or destructive noise apparatus which not only reduces noise, but also permits better communication between the operator and the patient.

Radio-frequency fields

Exposure to radio frequency occurs during MR examinations as the hydrogen nuclei are subjected to an oscillating magnetic field. The source of this electromagnetic radiation is the radio-frequency coils that surround the patient inside the magnet bore. 180° RF pulses use four times the power of a 90° RF pulse. For this reason fast spin echo sequences give the greatest concern for RF effects as they use a train of 180° RF pulses.

Radio-frequency irradiation

As the energy level of frequencies used in clinical MR imaging is relatively low and non-ionising compared with X-rays, visible light and microwaves, the predominant biological effect of RF irradiation absorption is the potential heating of tissue. Although non-thermal effects have been reported, they have not as yet been confirmed. As an excitation pulse is applied, some nuclei absorb the RF energy and enter the high energy state. As they relax, nuclei give off this absorbed energy to the surrounding lattice. In frequencies below 100 MHz, 90% of absorbed energy results from tissue currents (eddy currents in tissues), induced by the magnetic component of the radio frequency field. As frequency is increased, absorbed energy is also increased, therefore heating of tissue is largely frequency dependent. For this reason, RF heating is less of a concern in MR systems operating below 1.0 T.

Specific absorption rate (SAR)

The FDA limit for RF exposure is measured as either an increase in body temperature or as the specific absorption rate (SAR). The FDA limit for temperature is an increase of 1°C in the core of the body. In the periphery, higher increases to 38°C in the head, 39°C in the trunk and 40°C in the extremities are permitted. It is therefore necessary to measure RF absorption. This is manifested as tissue heating and the patient's ability to dissipate excess heat. RF absorption can be expressed in terms of SAR which in turn is expressed in Watts/kg, a quantity that depends on induced electric field, pulse duty cycle, tissue density, conductivity and the patient's size. Therefore the patient's weight and the pulse sequence parameters selected are important factors when monitoring SAR. Care must therefore be taken in recording the patient's proper weight to ensure the SAR does not exceed the permitted levels. SAR can be used to calculate an expected increase in body temperature during an average examination.

In the US, the recommended SAR level for imaging is 0.4 W/kg (whole body), 3.2 W/kg (head) and 8 W/kg (small volume). In Canada, the recommended SAR level is 2 W/kg. Recently, the FDA has reclassified MRI facilities. Sites that are studying the safety of scanning at SAR values above 4 W/kg whole body average are no longer required to limit their capabilities for proton imaging. Sites using research software may still require approval. The FDA also permits an attenuate criterion relying on temperature of the tissues. This is what most sites adhere to. For non-investigational MR sites, new modifications have been established to allow more slices per scan on body imaging. The FDA has acknowledged MR as an established diagnostic tool with recognised risks, that are well controlled by the design and use of the equipment.

Studies show that patient exposure up to ten times the recommended levels produces no serious adverse effects, despite elevations in skin and body temperatures. As body temperature increases, blood pressure and heart rate also increase slightly. Even though these effects seem insignificant, patients with compromised thermo-regulatory systems, may not be candidates for MR. In addition, those areas of the body with an inability to dissipate heat (the orbits and the testicles) have been evaluated independently, and in standard pulse sequences have shown no significant increase in temperature. Corneal temperatures were shown to increase from 0° to 1.8°C. However as some faster imaging sequences are developed which increase RF deposition to the patient, these areas may need to be re-evaluated.

RF antennae effects

Radio frequency fields can be responsible for significant burn hazards due to electrical currents that are produced in conductive loops. Equipment used in MRI, such as ECG leads and surface coils, should therefore be used with extreme caution. When using a surface coil, the operator must be careful to prevent any electrically conductive material (i.e. cable of surface coil), from forming a 'conductive loop' with itself or with the patient. Tissue or clothing could be potentially ignited by uninsulated cables. Coupling of a transmitting coil to a receive coil may also cause severe thermal injury. Routine checks of surface coils by the site's engineer should be performed to ensure proper function. It was recommended by the New York Academy of Science at a conference in which they presented 'Biological Effects and Safety Aspects of NMR', that wires used in MR imaging systems should be electrically and thermally insulated.

Claustrophobia

Although claustrophobia does not seem to be a safety issue, it is a condition that commonly affects patients and which MR operators should appreciate. RF heating, gradient noise and the confines of the magnet itself, add to the possibility of claustrophobic reactions.

Although the majority of these effects are transient, there have been two reported cases of patients who did not suffer from claustrophobia prior to the MR examination, but who not only had great difficulty in completing the examination, but also developed persistent claustrophobia. These patients required long term psychiatric treatment. Therefore, it is important to try to reduce the incidence of claustrophobia.

Controllable air movement within the bore of the magnet along with good patient contact and education, should help reduce claustrophobic reactions.

Quenching

Quenching is the process whereby there is a sudden loss of absolute zero of temperature in the magnet coils, so that they cease to be super conducting and become resistive. This results in helium escaping from the cryogen bath extremely rapidly. It may happen accidently or can be manually instigated in the case of an emergency. Quenching may cause severe and irreparable damage to the super conducting coils, and so a manual quench should only be performed in extreme cases when the physician and service engineer are involved in the decision to quench. A fire in the scan room may also be a cause to quench the magnet, so that fire fighting personnel can safely enter the room. All systems should have helium venting equipment, which removes the helium to the outside environment in the event of a quench. However if this fails, helium will vent into the room and replace the oxygen. For this reason, all scan rooms should contain an oxygen monitor that sounds an alarm if the oxygen falls below a certain level. Under these circumstances immediate evacuation of the patient and personnel is necessary. It should be noted that if the scan room door is closed when a quench occurs and helium escapes into the scan room, the depletion of oxygen causes a critical increase in pressure in the room compared with the control area. This produces high pressure in the scan room which may prevent opening of the door. This should only occur several minutes after a quench but if it does happen, the glass partition between the scan and control rooms should be broken to release the pressure. The scan room door can then be opened as usual and the patient evacuated. In such a case the patient should be immediately evacuated and evaluated for asphyxia, hypothermia and ruptured eardrums.

Safety education

Patient and personnel screening is the most effective way in which to avoid potential safety hazards to patients. Patients and MR employees with questionable ferromagnetic foreign objects either in or on their bodies, should be rigorously examined to avoid any serious health risks and accidents. Maintaining this controlled environment can be achieved by careful questioning and education of patients and all personnel. This is usually achieved via a screening questionnaire that is completed by all persons entering the magnetic field. The ISMRM has published a questionnaire that should be used as a guideline for screening forms. This must include patients, those accompanying patients for their examinations, staff and visitors.

Patient monitoring

It is recommended by the ISMRM Safety Committee that all patients are monitored 'verbally and visually'. Patients who cannot be contacted verbally and visually require more rigorous monitoring by pulse oximetry. These patients include those who are not responsive, those who are comatose, unconscious, sedated or hearing impaired, those who have weak voices or speak another language and paediatric patients.

Monitors and devices in MRI

There are specific criteria by which ancillary devices are deemed MR compatible. Such criteria recommended by the ISMRM include:

- FDA approval,
- FDA approval,
- manufacturer declaration,
- prior testing.

It is probably prudent to *trust no one* and test each device yourself before risking patient safety.
(There now follows a few tips for maintaining a safe, anxious free environment for the patients and their relatives.)

Safety tips

- Before sending the patient an appointment, check with them or the referring clinician, that they do not have a pacemaker or other contraindicated implants.
- Try to ascertain whether they are likely to suffer from claustrophobia as forearmed is forewarned! However, be careful how you question the

patient – mere suggestion of claustrophobia may create the problem itself!

- When sending out the appointment include any relevant safety information and details of the examination. Most of a patient's anxiety is fear of the unknown.
- Try to ensure that the waiting area is calming and pleasant.
- Carefully screen the patient and anyone else accompanying the patient into the scan room. This should include questions about surgical procedures, metal injury to the eye and pacemakers.
- Ensure that the patient and relatives/friends remove all credit cards, loose metal items, keys, jewellery, etc.
- Check for body piercing (any body part can be pierced!).
- Tattoos can heat up during image acquisition. A cool wet cloth placed over the tattoo acts as a good heat dissipater. Tattooed eyeliner may be contraindicated as heat can cause ocular damage.
- Bras and belts should also be removed even if they are non-ferrous and are not in the imaging field. They may still heat up and reduce image quality by locally altering the magnetic field.
- It is advisable to ask the patient to change into a gown for all examinations as this is really the only way of ensuring that the patient has removed all dangerous objects.
- The radiographer must always re-check the patient before they are taken into the magnetic field, regardless of how many times they have been checked before. It is the radiographer's responsibility to keep the MR environment safe. Remember, patients know nothing about magnetism and the potential hazards. Never trust them to check everything – always re-assess the patient before they are taken into the room. Anxious and sick patients especially cannot be trusted to give you correct information. Be extra vigilant with these types of patients. If you are in any doubt about their safety DO NOT TAKE THEM INTO THE MAGNETIC FIELD.
- Dealing with claustrophobic patients is a real art and every radiographer, nurse and radiologist has their own way of coaxing a patient into the magnet. Here are a few suggestions.
- The use of a mirror so that the patient can see out of the magnet often helps.
- Examining the patient prone when using the body coil can be very advantageous.
- Removing the pillow so that the patient's face is further away from the roof of the bore can help.
- Getting the patient to close their eyes or placing a piece of paper towel over their face may do the trick.
- Telling the patient that they do not have to have the examination and that although MR may be the best way of sorting out their problem, it is by no means the only way, gives the patient a feeling of control over their own destiny. It is astonishing how many times these few words have worked!

- Bringing the patient out of the magnet in between each sequence may help them to cope, especially in long procedures.
- Telling them that the magnet is open at both ends and that they are not shut in can be very reassuring.
- Use the bore light, the air circulation fan and the patient alarm system wherever possible.
- Encourage a relative or friend to accompany them and to maintain physical contact with them throughout the examination. The radiographer should always communicate with the patient during the examination to check that they are OK, and informing them of the length of pulse sequence. Also remember to tell them what is happening in-between sequences – there is nothing worse than lying in the magnet and thinking that everyone has gone home and left you.

Site planning

There are many difficult decisions to be made when installing a magnet system and careful consideration of these before a magnet is purchased, prevents unnecessary expenditure and wastage. Firstly, there are architectural requirements which include:

(1) structural reinforcement,
(2) spatial dimensions,
(3) mechanical and electrical components.

The decision to house the system in an existing building or whether a new building has to be constructed, is the primary consideration as the cost implications are quite considerable. Very often the field strength of the magnet is a limiting factor. At present, there are no real guidelines for determining the optimal field strength. Each facility has to evaluate the purpose of the system, and along with the local site considerations, decide on the field strength required. For example 0.5 T is probably adequate for imaging purposes, whereas at least 1.5 T is necessary if spectroscopy is to be carried out. The field strength is important because the size of the fringe field increases at higher field strengths. Shielding can control this, but also adds significantly to the cost of the unit.

The magnetic safety of personnel, equipment and structures and monitors outside the unit must be considered. The static field is three dimensional and extends above and below the magnet as well as to the sides. The magnetic field strength decreases with the cube of the distance from magnet, and any monitoring and computer devices should be located beyond the 5 G line. In addition, the entrance to the unit as well as the area surrounding the building must be free from magnetic field effects, to avoid people with pacemakers inadvertently walking into the field. Walls built around the building usually suffice.

Mobile MR units located in trucks have additional headaches. They must comply with road traffic regulations such as weight and wheel base area, as well as having a very restricted fringe field. For this reason most mobile units are 0.5 T or below. Some high field mobile systems can be ramped down for relocation. In addition, the site where the truck is parked must be level and strong enough to take the standing weight of the truck and its contents.

At any site, cooling and air conditioning requirements for the computer and its components should be assessed. Helium venting in the event of a quench, power supply and adequate door and room dimensions need to be taken into account. Adequate RF shielding should be installed and checks made to ensure that monitors and computers located in the vicinity do not interfere with the image. The floor plan of the scan room and the control room should be designed so that there can be rapid straight line evacuation to an area where emergency equipment can function properly. In short, the entire facility should be designed with the safety of the patients and personnel in mind. Magnetically controlled security doors located at all entrances to the magnetic field are often the best way of achieving this. In addition, routine preventative maintenance checks by the service engineer and continuing education is important. Therefore, careful planning and diligent upkeep of an MR facility can provide a safe environment for both patients and employees.

Questions

1. Which of the following's predominant biological effect is the heating of tissue?
   (a) static magnetic fields
   (b) time varying magnetic fields
   (c) radio frequency fields
   (d) all of the above.

2. The FDA limit for static main fields for clinical imaging is:
   (a) 1 G/cm
   (b) 6 T/s
   (c) up to 2 T
   (d) 1.5 T.

3. The general public should be restricted to:
   (a) 2 T and below
   (b) 20 T/s
   (c) 0.6 G
   (d) 5 G.

4. The reversible biological effect of static fields below 2 T is:
   (a) magnet haemodynamic effects
   (b) mild cutaneous sensation
   (c) stimulation of retinal phosphenes
   (d) increased body temperature.

5. The force with which a projectile approaches the magnet is influenced by:
   (a) gradient strength and rise time
   (b) the mass of the object and the distance from the magnet
   (c) the RF coil used
   (d) SAR.

6. RF antenna effects can cause:
   (a) better reception on your car radio
   (b) Rf interference artefacts
   (c) thermal injury
   (d) flames.

7. To evaluate patients for intra-ocular foreign bodies, it is recommended to use:
   (a) CT
   (b) one plain radiograph
   (c) your best judgement
   (d) two radiographic views.

8. The ISMRM Safety Committee recommends that pregnant employees in the MR environment:
   (a) may enter the scan room but should not remain while the scan is in progress
   (b) should not enter the scan room until after the first trimester
   (c) should work in CT
   (d) may enter the scan room and remain while the scan is in progress.

9. Complete the sentence. ... pulse sequences are of greater concern for RF effects whereas ... pulse sequences are of greater concern for TVMF.
   (a) Spin echo/gradient echo
   (b) Fast spin echo/EPI
   (c) EPI/fast spin echo
   (d) none of the above.

Chapter 11 Contrast Agents in MRI

Introduction

In previous chapters it has been discussed that multiple imaging acquisitions are required to adequately evaluate the patient. Clinical MRI typically utilises T1 weighted images with high intrinsic SNR to evaluate anatomy, and T2 weighted images with low SNR and high intrinsic contrast to evaluate pathology.

- On T1 weighted images, tissues with short T1 relaxation times (fat) appear bright and tissues with long T1 relaxation times (water) appear dark.
- On T2 weighted images, tissues with short T2 decay times (fat) appear dark and tissues with long T2 decay times (water) appear bright.

Since water demonstrates high signal intensity on T2 weighted images and tumours have a high content of free water, T2 weighted images are used to evaluate such lesions. However, there are pathological conditions in which the high intrinsic contrast provided by T2 weighted images, may be insufficient to detect lesions accurately. Furthermore, although SNR is increased in T1 weighted images, the majority of lesions are inconspicuous because both water and tumours demonstrate low signal intensities. In order to increase contrast between pathology and normal tissue, enhancement agents may be introduced that selectively affect the T1 and T2 relaxation times in these tissues. This chapter discusses the clinical applications, methodology, administration and precautions of several different enhancement agents used in MRI.

Uses and methodology

It has been clearly shown that enhancement agents are valuable in detecting tumours, infection, infarction, inflammation, and post-traumatic lesions in the central nervous system (CNS) and in the body. There are MR enhancement agents that affect the T1 and/or T2 relaxation times of different tissues thereby introducing a contrast difference. The way in which this occurs is best understood by reviewing the basic principles of weighting in MRI.

Review of weighting

There are several parameters that influence inherent image contrast. These include those over which there is no control, and those which can be controlled. The extrinsic parameters which can be controlled in order to acquire the MR image include:

(1) pulse sequence type (spin echo, inversion recovery and gradient echo),
(2) TR,
(3) TE,
(4) TI,
(5) flip angle.

Parameters which previously could not be controlled are:

(1) T1 recovery time,
(2) T2 decay time,
(3) relative proton density within the tissue.

Proton density

The proton density is the relative amount of mobile water and fat protons available within the sample of tissue that is being imaged. Proton density is responsible for the initial amplitude of the signal or the height of the FID. In MRI since TR controls T1 weighting and TE controls T2 weighting the effects of proton density on the images is manipulated by selecting a TR longer than the T1 recovery time of most tissues (more than 2000 ms), and a TE shorter than the T2 decay time of the majority of tissues (less than 20 ms). This results in proton density weighted images, where tissues with high proton densities such as CSF, tumours and fat, appear bright.

T2 decay

T2 relaxation occurs as a loss of phase coherence among proton spins. After the RF pulse is withdrawn, nuclei are in phase with each other (coherent). Since the magnetic field strength experienced by the nuclei determines their precessional frequency, changes in B_0 and local inhomogeneities alter the individual precessional frequencies of the nuclei causing them to dephase. This reduces their T2 decay times and as dephasing increases, the signal intensity decreases as there is less coherent magnetisation present in the transverse plane. To exploit this effect, a short TE is selected to minimise T2 weighting and a long TE is selected to maximise it.

In MRI since TE controls T2 weighting the effect of T2 decay in the images is manipulated by selecting a TR longer than the T1 recovery time of most tissues (more than 2000 ms), and a TE during the time in which T2 decay is occurring in the majority of tissues (more than 80 ms). This results in a T2 weighted image where tissues with long T2 relaxation times (water and tumour) appear bright, and tissues with short T2 times appear dark (fat).

T1 recovery

T1 recovery is the longitudinal recovery of the NMV. Before the RF excitation pulse is applied, some magnetic moments are said to be in thermal equilibrium as more nuclei align parallel with the field (low energy state), than oppose the field (high energy state). The NMV which represents the sum of the magnetic moments is therefore parallel to B_0. During RF pulse excitation, some nuclei absorb transmitted RF energy and enter the high energy state. The resultant sum of the magnetic moments causes the NMV to lie in the transverse plane. After the withdrawal of the RF pulse some high energy nuclei transfer their absorbed energy and return to the low energy state. As this occurs, the NMV returns to its original orientation parallel to B_0 and so recovers longitudinally. To exploit this effect the TR is selected to control the amount of longitudinal recovery permitted between excitation pulses. Short TRs maximise T1 weighting, longer TRs minimise it.

In MRI, since TR controls T1 weighting the effect of T1 recovery in the images is manipulated by selecting a TR during the time in which T1 recovery time is occurring in most tissues (less than 1000 ms), and TE shorter than the T2 decay time of the majority of tissues (less than 20 ms). The result is a T1 weighted image where tissues with short T1 times appear bright (fat), and tissues with long T1 relaxation times (water and tumours) appear dark.

Mechanism of action

Both T1 recovery and T2 decay are influenced by the magnetic field experienced locally within the nucleus. The local magnetic field responsible for these processes is caused by:

(1) the main magnetic field,
(2) the fluctuations caused by the magnetic moments of nuclear spins in neighbouring molecules.

These molecules *rotate* or *tumble*, and the rate of rotation of the molecules is a characteristic property of the solution. It is dependent upon:

(1) the viscosity of the solution,
(2) the temperature of the solution.

Both T1 and T2 recovery times can be changed by the introduction of contrast agents. Some agents primarily shorten T1 and some shorten T2. When the predominant effect is T1 shortening, structures with a reduced T1 relaxation time appear bright on T1 weighted images. When the predominant effect is T2 shortening, structures with a reduced T2 relaxation time appear dark on T2 weighted images. The former are known as T1 agents and the latter as T2 agents. These effects are now described in more detail.

At magnetic field strengths commonly used in MRI, the speed of the molecular rotation is closely matched to the precessional frequency of the nuclei. As molecules tumble, magnetic moments within the molecules have varying effects on the externally applied magnetic field, and ultimately the field experienced by the nucleus. In Fig. 11.1, the tumbling or rotation of the magnetic moments of hydrogen in water molecules is illustrated.

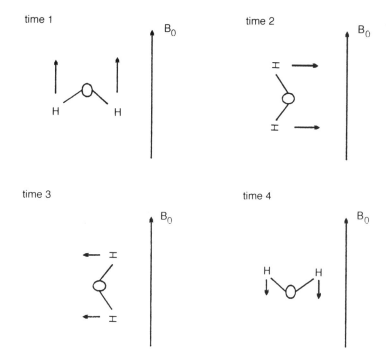

Fig. 11.1 Tumbling of water molecules.

During time 1, the magnetic moments of the hydrogen nuclei add to B_0, during times 2 and 3 there is no net effect as the magnetic moments lie perpendicular to B_0, and at time 4 they impose a negative effect on the applied field B_0. This tumbling therefore results in local fluctuations in the magnetic field. Molecules that tumble with a frequency at or near the Larmor frequency, have more efficient T1 recovery times than other molecules. Therefore, when local magnetic field fluctuations occur at or near the Larmor frequency of hydrogen, the T1 relaxation time of hydrogen is reduced.

Dipole-dipole interactions

The phenomenon by which excited protons are affected by nearby excited protons and electrons is called dipole–dipole interaction. Water within the body tumbles much faster than the Larmor frequency, resulting in inefficient relaxation and a long T1 relaxation time. If a tumbling molecule with a large magnetic moment is placed in the presence of water protons, local magnetic field fluctuations occur. Molecular tumbling creates fluctuations in a magnetic field near the Larmor frequency, and so T1 relaxation times of nearby protons can be reduced. This is the effect that occurs when enhancement agents that have large magnetic moments come into contact with water protons – the T1 relaxation times of the protons is reduced so they appear bright (not dark) on a T1 weighted image. In addition, when a substance that demonstrates high positive magnetic susceptibility comes into contact with tissues with long T2 decay times, they too can be reduced so they appear dark (not bright) on T2 weighted images.

Magnetic susceptibility

When evaluating suitable enhancement agents, their magnetic suscept-ibility must be considered. Magnetic susceptibility is a fundamental property of matter and is defined as the ability of the external magnetic field to affect the nucleus of an atom and magnetise it. Magnetic susceptibility effects include diamagnetism, paramagnetism and ferro-magnetism. As discussed in Chapter 9:

- Diamagnetic substances such as gold and silver show mild negative effects on the local magnetic field within the nucleus.
- Paramagnetic substances such as gadolinium chelates have a positive effect on the local magnetic field.
- Super-paramagnetic substances have large magnetic moments and create large disruptive changes in local magnetic fields.
- Ferromagnetic substances such as iron acquire large magnetic moments when placed in a magnetic field and retain this magnetisation even when the external field is removed.

T1 agents

As paramagnetic substances have positive magnetic susceptibilities, they provide a suitable choice for an enhancement agent in MRI. *Gadolinium*

(Gd), a trivalent lanthanide element, is ideal because it has seven unpaired electrons and an ability to allow rapid exchange of bulk water. Water within the body (such as that found in tumours), tumbles much faster than the Larmor frequency, resulting in inefficient relaxation that is demonstrated by long T1 and T2 relaxation times. If a substance with a large magnetic moment (such as gadolinium) is placed in the presence of tumbling water protons, fluctuations in the local magnetic field are created. When molecular tumbling creates fluctuations in a magnetic field near the Larmor frequency, the T1 relaxation times of nearby water protons can be reduced. This results in an increased signal intensity of these protons on T1 weighted images. For this reason, gadolinium is known as a *T1 enhancement agent*.

T2 agents

Paramagnetic agents have been used effectively for several years however there are super-paramagnetic agents that can be used as T2 enhancement agents. In order to increase contrast in a specific tissue, an area must be either brighter or darker than the surrounding structures. Substances such as iron oxides can be used to shorten the T2 decay times and thus decrease signal intensity on T2 weighted images. Iron oxides shorten relaxation times of nearby hydrogen atoms and therefore reduce the signal intensity in normal tissues. This results in a signal loss on proton density weighted or heavily T2 weighted images. For this reason super-paramagnetic iron oxides are known as *T2 enhancement agents*. One such agent is Feridex™ I.V.

Relaxivity

When contrast agents are used in computed tomography (CT), the enhancement is due to concentrations of the agent. When contrast agents are used in MRI it is not the agent itself but the effects of the agent that is measured.

The effect of a substance on relaxation rate is known as its *relaxivity*. As previously discussed, water tumbles much faster than the Larmor frequency resulting in inefficient relaxation and persistence of phase coherence. T1 and T2 times are directly affected by local magnetic fields and any substance that affects T1 also affects T2 as they do not occur independently of one another. Since short T1 and long T2 relaxation times both increase signal intensity, it would seem difficult to find a substance that both shortens the T1 time and lengthens the T2 time. Relaxivity is expressed in the following equation where

$$(1/T1)\text{observed} = (P)\,(1/T1)\text{enhanced} + (1-P)\,(1/T1)\text{bulk water}$$

and

$$(1/T2)\text{observed} = (P)\,(1/T2)\text{enhanced} + (1-P)\,(1/T2)\text{bulk water}$$

The relaxivity equation shows that the inverse of T1 in bulk water combined with an enhancement agent results in a new relaxivity, (1/T)enhanced. *P* is the fraction or concentration of the substance, and therefore as the concentration is increased the effect of the agent is also increased. The equation also demonstrates that T1 and T2 are equally affected by enhancement agents. However, since the T2 relaxation time of biological fluids (approximately 100 ms) is much shorter then the T1 relaxation time (approximately 2000 ms), a higher effective concentration of the enhancement agent is needed to produce significant shortening of T2.

As the static magnetic field B_0 is responsible for altering the precessional frequency of protons bound to different sites on the molecule, it produces an effect (previously described) known as chemical shift. Chemical shift increases as the magnitude of B_0 increases. Substances such as gadolinium do not affect the static magnetic field and subsequently have little effect on chemical shift. Therefore at recommended doses gadolinium has the greatest effect on altering T1 relaxation times. However, substances such as iron oxides do affect the static magnetic field and thus the precessional frequencies of individual nuclei. This results in an increase in dephasing and a shortening of T2 decay times. These agents are known as *selective T2 agents*. It should be noted that the relaxivity equation assumes no chemical shift and so a chemical exchange broadening term must be added in order to evaluate iron oxides accurately.

Gadolinium safety

Gadolinium is a rare earth metal (lanthanide) more commonly known as a 'heavy metal'. Metal ions with free electrons tend to accumulate in tissues with a natural affinity for metals (*binding sites*). Sites within the body that bind Gd^{+3} include membranes, transport proteins, enzymes, and the osseous matrix (lungs, liver, spleen, and bone). As the body is unable to excrete these metals, they can remain for a long period of time.

Fortunately there are substances with a high affinity for metal ions. These substances are known as *chelates*. The chelate (meaning claw in Greek), binds some of the available sites of the metal ion. A commonly used chelate is *diethylene triaminepentaacetic acid (DTPA)*. DTPA binds eight of the nine binding sites of the gadolinium ion leaving the ninth free for close approach of water molecules to the paramagnetic centre. By binding the rare earth metal ion gadolinium, with the chelate DTPA (a ligand), *Gd-DTPA* (gadopentetate) is formed. It is a relatively safe, water soluble contrast enhancement agent for MRI. The gadopentetate molecule has two negative charges that must be balanced in solution by two positively charged meglumine ions, and it is therefore ionic. Another agent that received FDA approval is *Gd-HP-DO3A* (gadoteridol) in which the charges have been balanced to produce a non-ionic contrast agent. The structure of the *HP-DO3A* ligand differs from that of DTPA as it is macrocyclic, affording greater stability and a reduced tendency for release of the toxic gadolinium atom. Other chelates soon to be available include *Gd-DTPA-BMA (gadodiamide)*, a non-ionic derivative of *Gd-DTPA*, and *GdDOTA*, an ionic macrocyclic molecule (Fig. 11.2).

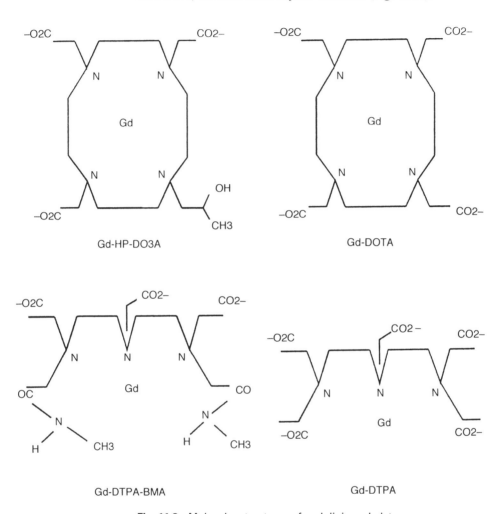

Fig. 11.2 Molecular structures of gadolinium chelates.

Gadolinium side effects and contraindications

At standard doses the side effects of gadolinium chelates are minimal when compared with those of iodinated contrast agents that can cause anaphylaxis and even death. Studies show that the side effects associated with gadopentetate dimeglumine include:

(1) a slight transitory increase in bilirubin and blood iron,
(2) 9.8% mild transitory headaches,

(3) 4.1% nausea,
(4) 2% vomiting,
(5) less than 1% hypotension gastrointestinal upset or rash.

At present, there have been two reported cases (out of 500 000 injections) of death attributed to the introduction of gadolinium into the body. Approximately 80% of gadolinium is excreted by the kidneys in three hours and 98% is recovered by faeces and urine in one week. Although there are no known contraindications for the use of gadolinium at this time, there are several situations where caution should be used before administering gadolinium, these include haematological disorders such as haemolytic anaemia, sickle cell anaemia, pregnancy, lactating mothers, respiratory disorders, asthma and previous allergic history.

Gadolinium administration

The effective dosage of Gd-DTPA and Gd-DTPA-BMA is 0.1 millimoles per kilogram of body weight (mmol/kg), (0.2 ml/kg or approximately 0.1 ml/lb), with a maximum dose of 20 ml. Gd-HP-DO3A has been approved for up to 0.3 mmol/kg or three times the dose of Gd-DTPA. The lethal dose, determined in rat studies is never approached in the clinical situation and is 10 mmol/kg. This is a similar safety factor to the 400 mg/kg effective and the 6000 mg/kg lethal dose of iodine.

Feridex™ safety

Feridex™ is a super-paramagnetic iron oxide with dextran for intravenous administration. Chemically, ferrous oxide is a non-stoichiometric magnetic. The iron in Feridex™ enters the normal body iron metabolism demonstrated by a transient increase in serum iron values one day after injection and increased serum ferritin values seven days after administration.

Feridex™ side effects and contraindications

Adverse side effects occur in less than 5% of the population that receive the agent. These include mild to severe back, leg and groin pain and in a few cases, head and neck pain. In clinical trials, 2.5% of subjects experienced pain severe enough to cause interruption or discontinuation of the drug. A few patients experience digestive side effects including nausea, vomiting and diarrhoea. Anaphylactic-like reactions and hypotension have been reported in a few patients receiving Feridex™. Feridex™ is contraindicated in patients with known allergies/hypersensitivity to iron, parenteral dextran, parenteral iron-dextran or parenteral iron-polysaccaride preparations. After administration of the contrast agent, full resuscitation facilities should be available. In addition, since the infusion is dark in colour, skin surrounding the infusion site might discolour if there is extravasation. For more information see the package insert of Feridex®.

Feridex® administration

The recommended dose of Feridex® iron oxide is 0.56 mg of iron (0.05 ml Feridex® I.V.) per kg of body weight. This should be diluted in 100 ml of 50% dextrose and given intravenously over 30 min. The diluted drug is administered through a 5 micron filter at a rate of 2–4 mm per min. This agent should be used within 8 hours following dilution.

Current applications of contrast agents

Gadolinium has proven invaluable in imaging the central nervous system because of its ability to pass through breakdowns in the blood–brain barrier (BBB). Clinical indications for the head, spine and body for gadolinium include:

(1) tumours pre- and post-operation,
(2) pre- and post-radiotherapy,
(3) infection,
(4) infarction,
(5) inflammation,
(6) post-traumatic lesions,
(7) post-operation lumbar disc.

Head and spine (Figs 11.3–11.9)

Extra axial areas or areas outside the BBB demonstrate normal enhancement. These areas include the falx, petrous matrix, choroid plexus, pineal gland, pituitary gland, and the infundibulum. The diagnosis of other extra-axial lesions such as acoustic neuromas and meningiomas has been facilitated by the use of gadolinium. Areas with slow flowing blood such as the cavernous sinus and the venous drainage system may also demonstrate enhancement. Therefore, fat and slow flowing blood can often be mistaken for blood products. In the pituitary gland a macro adenoma enhances rapidly but a micro adenoma, because of its densely packed cells, does not enhance and therefore appears dense compared with the normal enhancement of the sella tursica. Figures 11.3 to 11.5 show images of the brain pre- and post-gadolinium injection.

Intra-axial lesions such as infarcts and tumours enhance due to the breakdown in their BBB, but peri-infarctal oedema does not enhance. Although recent infarctions do not enhance until the BBB has been disrupted, some evidence suggests that arterial vessels in the brain

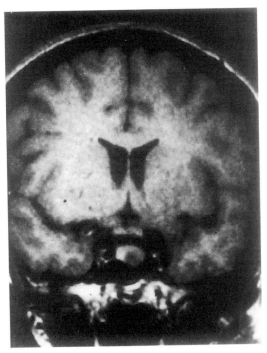 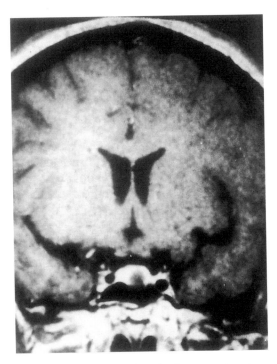

Fig. 11.3 Coronal T1 weighted spin echo images of the brain pre- and post-gadolinium injection. On the enhanced image (right) an area within the sella enhances but there is also an area of low signal intensity. This indicates a pituitary micro-adenoma.

enhance and therefore any occlusion or slow flow in these vessels can be demonstrated (Fig. 11.6).

Metastatic disease can be demonstrated with the use of gadolinium. Studies have shown that at higher doses metastatic lesions are more conspicuous. As patient management often changes according to the number of intra-cranial metastases demonstrated, the ability to demonstrate these lesions can be important.

Spinal cord lesions may also be well visualised with the use of gadolinium. Although lesions can sometimes be detected without the use of gadolinium, in some cases circumscribing the lesion with enhancement agents can demonstrate the presence of other anomalies such as a syrinx. Lesions such as MS and other infectious disorders such as AIDS and abscesses, also enhance with the use of gadolinium (Fig. 11.7). Enhancing MS plaques may indicate activity within the plaque.

Perfusion is micro-circulation or the delivery of blood to tissues. Perfusion imaging is the measurement of blood volume in these areas. This measurement however is complicated because less than 5% of tissue protons are intravascular. To measure perfusion the signal intensity in perfusing spins may be suppressed or increased. This can be achieved by either employing motion sensitive gradients (as in diffusion imaging), or by introducing enhancement agents. Agents like gadolinium and iron oxide

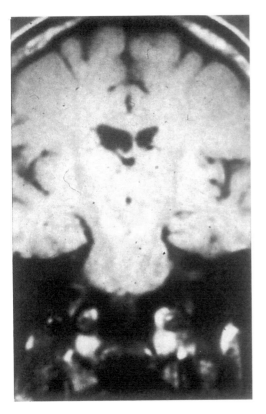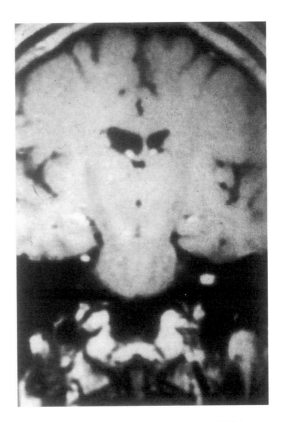

Fig. 11.4 Coronal T1 weighted images of the head pre- and post-gadolinium injection. On the enhanced image (right) an area within the internal auditory meatus has enhanced. This indicates an acoustic neuroma. There is also a tiny enhancing lesion on the fifth cranial nerve.

may be localised in the capillary bed and produce large magnetic moments in the capillary network, creating magnetic fields that extend into the adjacent tissues. This results in perfusion information in patients with ischaemia in brain parenchyma, liver parenchyma and in myocardial infarction.

Subtle enhancement can be shown in the scar in post-operative discectomy patients when differentiating between scar tissue and recurrent herniated disc – scar enhances and disc does not. However, after approximately 30 min, disc matter shows signs of enhancement. For this reason, it is advisable to scan immediately after injection in cases where scar is suspected (Fig. 11.8).

Bone lesions of the spine can be well visualised with the use of gadolinium. However, some metastatic lesions of the spine appear as low signal intensities on T1 weighted images relative to the high signal intensities caused by fat in the bone marrow. Enhancement can raise the signal intensity of the bone lesion to that of normal marrow making the lesion iso-intense with normal bone (Fig. 11.9). Fat selective saturation

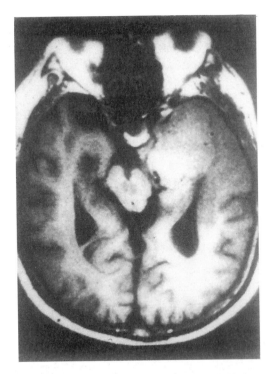
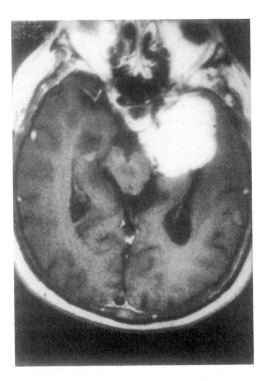

Fig. 11.5 Axial T1 weighted images of the brain pre- and post-gadolinium injection. On the enhanced image (right) enhancement of the peripheral temporal lobe is demonstrated. This indicates a meningioma.

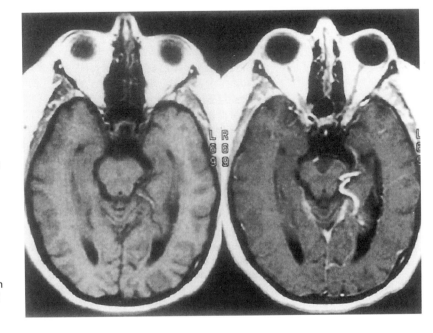

Fig. 11.6 These axial images of the brain were acquired before (left) and after (right) contrast enhancement. The slow flow in the arterio-venous malformation (AVM) demonstrates enhancement after contrast enhancement. The T2 and T2* weighted images for this case are given in Chapter 12 (Fig. 12.15) and can be compared.

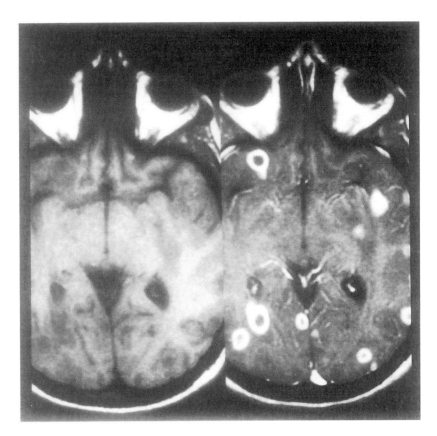

Fig. 11.7 Axial T1 weighted images pre- and post-injection of gadolinium. The ring enhancing lesions demonstrate toxoplasmosis in this 24-year-old male with AIDS.

pulses can be used to suppress fat marrow and so visualise enhancing lesions.

Body (Figs 11.10–11.16)

The use of gadolinium in body imaging is increasing. Even though contrast does not enhance all lesions within the body, gadolinium has shown some promising effects. Metastatic lesions of the bone have been more clearly delineated by the use of gadolinium. Since the liver, spleen and kidneys are vascular organs contrast enhances these structures almost immediately after injection. For this reason, rapid imaging is recommended (see Chapter 12). Dynamic enhancement and rapid imaging can be used to evaluate arterial flow in abdominal vessels by using 3D T1 gradient echo breath-hold acquisitions after gadolinium. Peak enhancement differences occur shortly after injection, and by two minutes after injection lesions begin to enhance so that they are iso-intense with normal organ parenchyma. For this reason, rapid imaging acquisitions should be used when imaging the abdomen to maximise the enhancement effect (Figs 11.10 and 11.11).

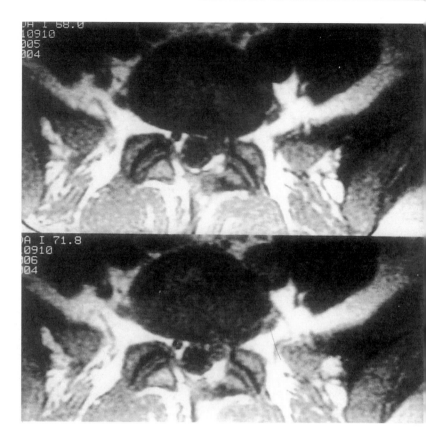

Fig. 11.8 Axial T1 weighted images of the lumbar spine pre and post gadolinium injection. The subtle enhancement posterior to the vertebral body and bulging out into the caudal sac demonstrates a recurrent disk wrapped in scar tissue.

In cardiac imaging, myocardial infarctions have been shown to enhance. Gadolinium has also been used for perfusion studies of the kidneys and some bladder lesions enhance on T1 weighted images. Most lesions in the abdomen, however, have been demonstrated quite adequately on T2 weighted sequences without the use of relaxation enhancing agents.

In breast imaging, the use of gadolinium followed by repeated rapid acquisition techniques is proving to help determine the nature of suspicious lesions within the breast tissue. In general many rapidly enhancing and/or spiculated enhanced lesions are thought to be malignant. In addition, this technique seems to demonstrate multi-focal lesions that are not always apparent on plain mammography (Fig. 11.12).

Figures 11.13–11.16 show further applications of gadolinium and Feridex® in the body.

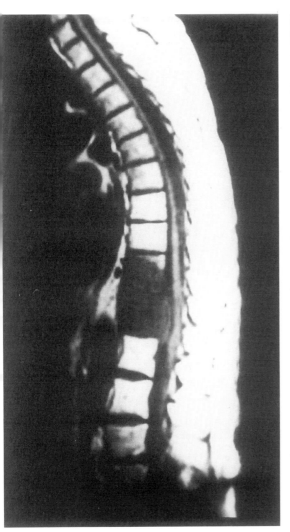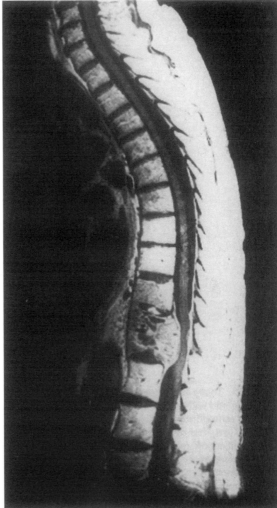

Fig. 11.9 Sagittal T1 weighted images of the thoracic spine pre- and post-gadolinium injection. The low signal intensity in the spine on the unenhanced image is an area of bone metastases. After enhancement the signal intensity is raised to that of normal bone.

Oral and rectal enhancement agents (Fig. 11.17)

Gastrointestinal contrast agents are not as widely used as intravascular agents at present but may increase in use in the future. Oral contrast agents have been researched for bowel enhancement. Iron oxides as well as fatty substances have been used orally to try to enhance effectively the gastrointestinal tract. However due to constant peristalsis, these agents enhance bowel motion artefacts more often than enhancing pathologic

(a)

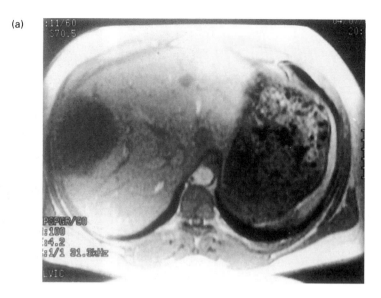

(b)

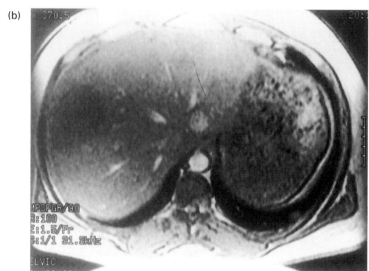

Fig. 11.10 These liver images were acquired with a fast gradient echo during breath hold and just after dynamic contrast injection. (a) demonstrates enhancement of liver parenchyma but little enhancement of the lesion. By the next acquisition (b) the liver and lesion both demonstrate enhancement and therefore become isointense.

lesions. The use of anti-spasmodic agents helps to retard peristalsis and/ or ultra-fast imaging techniques to decrease these artefacts. Some facilities have used blueberry juice and dilute gadolinium to enhance bowel. In addition, agents such as dilute barium solutions can be used to make bowel contents appear dark. Air has also been used as an effective contrast agent in the rectum. By showing a signal intensity void in the distended rectum, the prostate in males and the uterus in females can be more clearly demonstrated when imaging the pelvis (Fig. 11.17).

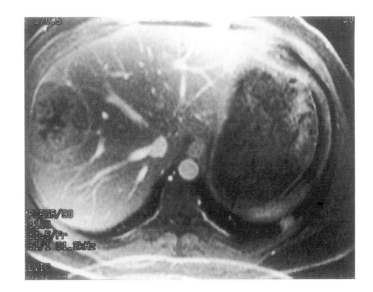

Fig. 11.11 This liver image was acquired with a fast gradient echo with fat suppression. Note that the lesion is now demonstrating ring enhancement on this delayed acquisition.

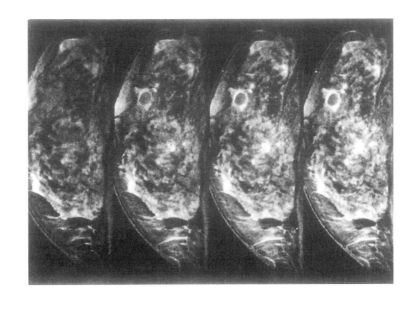

Fig. 11.12 These breast images were acquired with a fast gradient echo acquisition with fat suppression. Images were acquired before (far left), immediately after (28 s) (second from left), later (56 s) (second from right) and delayed (2 min) (far right) contrast injection. This lesion filled slowly and demonstrated a relatively smooth border and therefore was thought to be cystic and benign.

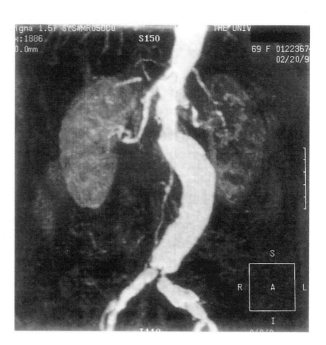

Fig. 11.13 This coronal image of the abdominal vessels was acquired with a 3D T1 fast gradient echo acquisition during breath-hold and dynamic injection of the double-dose gadolinium. Note the degree of renal artery stenosis demonstrated on this image.

Conclusion

Overall examination time may lengthen with the use of intravenous contrast in MRI as additional sequences are performed. In most cases T1 and T2 weighted sequences should be performed prior to the use of gadolinium followed by contrast and another T1 weighted series. Gadolinium has improved the visualisation of lesions in many cases and it has enabled a more precise delineation of lesions in T1 weighted images. It is also a safer form of enhancing agent than iodine and currently the most effective contrast agent in MRI.

The greatest effect of the increased use of enhancement agents has been on the system operator. The operator should be aware that contrast not only enhances lesions but also enhances slow flowing vessels. Flow motion artefacts increase with the use of gadolinium and should therefore be anticipated and compensated for by the operator especially when imaging vascular areas of the body. In addition, gadolinium should be used in conjunction with fat suppression techniques in areas where it is suspected that the increased signal from enhancement will become iso-intense with fatty tissues.

Lastly, different concentrations of gadolinium will affect image contrast and produce a layering effect in the bladder (Fig. 11.18).

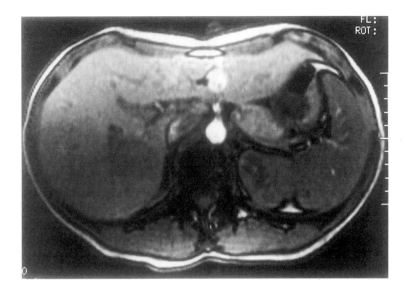

Fig. 11.14(a) This axial T1 gradient echo of the liver was acquired before contrast enhancement.

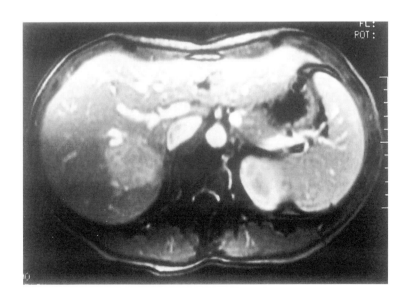

Fig. 11.14(b) This liver image was acquired with a fast T1 gradient echo after gadolinium enhancement. Because of arterial feeders, this lesion does enhance before normal liver parenchyma.

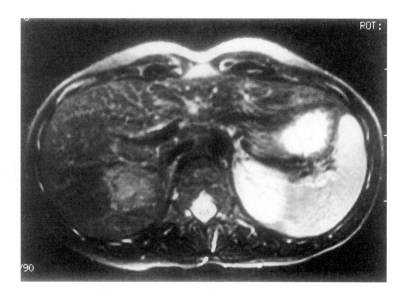

Fig. 11.15(a) This axial T2 fast spin echo was acquired before contrast enhancement.

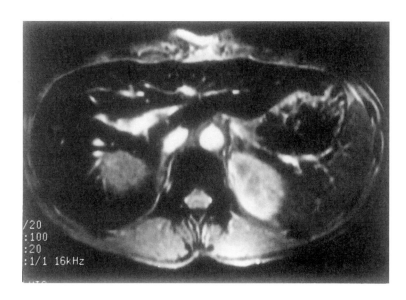

Fig. 11.15(b) This liver image was acquired with a fast T2 acquisition after an injection of Feridex®. Note that the normal portions of the liver are perfused by the agent and are black whereas the liver lesion remains somewhat unchanged by the iron oxide injection.

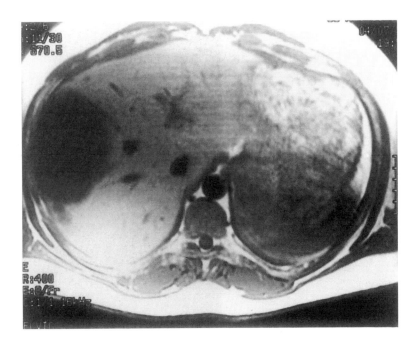

Fig. 11.16 This liver image was acquired with a spin echo T1 acquisition prior to contrast enhancement. Note the large liver lesion in the right lobe of the liver demonstrated as an area of low signal intensity.

Questions

1. Complete the sentence. Fluid filled lesions generally appear ... on T1 weighting and ... on T2 weighting.
   (a) hyperintenese/hyperintense
   (b) hypointense/hypointense
   (c) hyperintense/hypointense
   (d) hypointense/hyperintense.

2. Complete the sentence. Paramagnetic contrast agents have their primary effect on ... and are called ... agents.
   (a) T2/T1
   (b) T1/T1
   (c) T2/T2
   (d) T1/T2.

3. Are T1 or T2 relaxation times influenced by local magnetic fields?

4. Are gadolinium chelates diamagnetic, paramagnetic or ferromagnetic?

5. Precautions for Feridex™ use include:
   (a) hypersensitivity to iron
   (b) renal failure
   (c) pregnancy
   (d) all of the above.

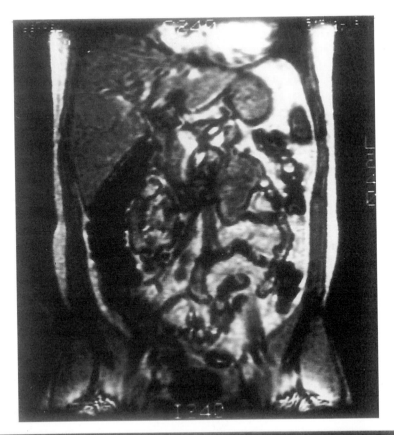

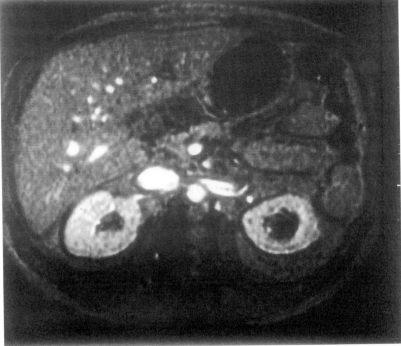

Fig. 11.17 Coronal and axial images using an incoherent RF spoiled gradient echo sequence with dilute barium solution. In both images low signal intensity is demonstrated in the stomach (axial) and bowel (coronal).

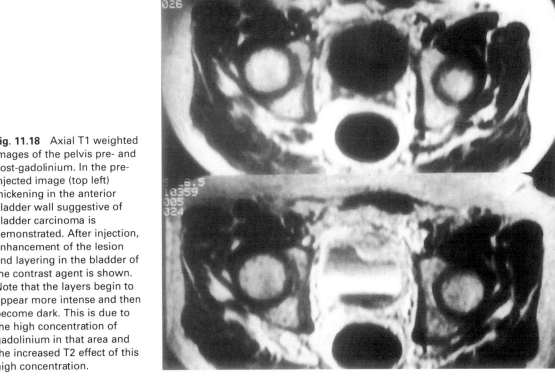

Fig. 11.18 Axial T1 weighted images of the pelvis pre- and post-gadolinium. In the pre-injected image (top left) thickening in the anterior bladder wall suggestive of bladder carcinoma is demonstrated. After injection, enhancement of the lesion and layering in the bladder of the contrast agent is shown. Note that the layers begin to appear more intense and then become dark. This is due to the high concentration of gadolinium in that area and the increased T2 effect of this high concentration.

6. Contraindications for gadolinium are:
   (a) renal failure
   (b) pregnancy
   (c) none known
   (d) a and b.

7. The recommended dose for gadolinium is:
   (a) 1.0 mmol/kg
   (b) 0.1 mmol/kg
   (c) 0.1 cc/kg
   (d) 0.2 mmol/kg.

8. Structures that normally enhance with gadolinium include:
   (a) the pituitary and the falx
   (b) corpus callosum and the basal ganglia
   (c) all tumours
   (d) only tumours.

9. When should rapid imaging techniques be considered with gadolinium enhancement?

Chapter 12   Advanced Imaging Techniques

Introduction

Pulse sequences have evolved rapidly over the relatively short life span of MRI. Pulse sequences such as conventional spin echo and inversion recovery provide excellent morphological images of the body, particularly structures undergoing little physiological motion. However, such sequences yield long scan and examination times, sometimes in the order of hours. Rapid imaging sequences such as fast spin echo and gradient echo have provided more acceptable scan times and higher resolution images but can still result in limited patient throughput and image artefacts due to patient motion.

The previous chapters introduce the basis for MRI by describing fundamental pulse sequences and image formation for spin echo, gradient echo, inversion recovery and fast spin echo, and presenting a brief introduction to EPI. Recent technical developments in system hardware and software have allowed for ultra-fast imaging sequences in the order of milliseconds. Although some ultra-fast sequences can be performed on conventional scanners, EPI, currently the fastest data acquisition strategy, requires specially designed hardware.

Ultra-fast imaging sequences permit an almost unlimited range of applications that were never possible with conventional MR imaging sequences. Such applications include:

- breath-hold imaging,
- functional brain imaging,
- perfusion and diffusion imaging,
- real-time imaging of cardiac motion and perfusion,
- fast abdominal imaging,
- improved MR angiography,
- real-time monitoring of interventional procedures.

This chapter will describe several recent developments in the mechanisms of advanced imaging techniques and their potential applications. Firstly, however, as most new sequences require upgraded hardware systems, developments in high speed gradients are now discussed.

High speed gradient systems

One of the greatest factors that affects the timing of a pulse sequence is gradient switching. During the sequence each of the three gradients (X,Y and Z) are switched on and off many times for spatial encoding and for signal refocusing (see Fig. 3.14). Each time a gradient is switched on, power is applied to the gradient until it reaches maximum amplitude. The gradient is then left on for a period of time and then reversed for the same period of time. The application of each gradient therefore represents 'dead time' and, as gradients are applied many times during the sequences, each millisecond of wasted time is multiplied for each acquisition. The sum of wasted seconds represents a considerable time loss resulting in longer TRs and TEs, shorter turbo factors, less imaging slices and longer scan times. Significant timesavings are therefore achievable by modifications to the gradient system. To investigate this, it is necessary to evaluate the main components of a balanced gradient system which include:

- *gradient amplitude* measured in millitesla per metre (mT/m) or gauss per centimetre (G/cm),
- *gradient rise time* measured in microseconds (µs),
- *slew rate* measured in millitesla per metre per second (mT/m/s),
- *duty cycle*, the percentage of time that the gradient is permitted to work.

Gradient amplitude

The strength of the gradient is known as the gradient amplitude. Gradient amplitudes vary but typical gradient strengths are 10 mT/m. This means that when the gradient has reached maximum amplitude its strength changes the magnetic field 10 mT over each metre or 1 gauss over each centimetre (10 mT/m = 1 G/cm) Gradient amplitudes directly affect image resolution as high gradient amplitudes are required for a small FOV and thin slices (Fig. 12.1).

Gradient rise time

The time that it takes for gradients to reach their maximum strength or amplitude is known as the gradient rise time (Fig. 12.1). If the rise time is reduced, time is saved within the pulse sequence which is then translated into shorter overall imaging times. High gradient amplitudes allow for

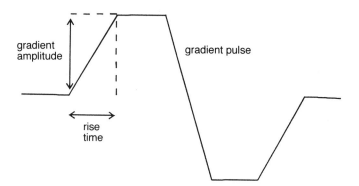

Fig. 12.1 Gradient amplitude versus rise time.

shorter rise times. As shown in Fig. 12.2, the application of enough power to create high gradient amplitudes shortens rise times but yields a power overshoot. In addition, high gradient amplitudes permit high amplitude balancing lobes allowing for timesavings within pulse sequences (this technique will be described in more detail later in this chapter). Therefore for ultra-fast and/or ultra-high resolution images, higher gradient amplitudes of 20 mT/m or greater are required.

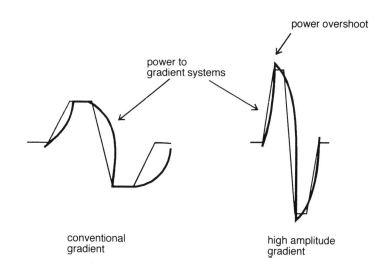

Fig. 12.2 Comparison of the power supply to conventional and high speed gradient systems.

Slew rate

The slew rate is describe as the strength of the gradient over distance. Typical gradient slew rates are in the order of 70 mT/m/s. High speed gradients are generally 120 mT/m/s. Some investigational slew rates approach 240 mT/m/s but at present this exceeds the FDA guidelines for gradient strength.

Duty cycle

This is a percentage of time during the TR period that the gradient is permitted to be at maximum amplitude, or to 'work', during an imaging sequence. This work time is known as the duty cycle. The duty cycle increases with slew rate but as the duty cycle increases, the number of attainable slices is reduced. In spin echo imaging the typical duty cycle is 10% whereas in EPI it is closer to 50% of the TR period.

Balanced gradient systems

In a balanced gradient system each gradient pulse is balanced by an equal but opposite gradient pulse. For example, a positive gradient pulse is followed by a negative pulse to, in effect, undo the changes caused by the positive lobe. Therefore, in a balanced gradient system, the area under the positive lobe of the gradient equals the area under the negative lobe (Fig. 12.3).

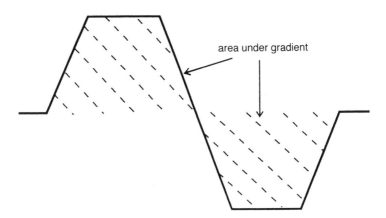

area under gradient

Fig. 12.3 Balanced gradients.

During readout, the amplitude of the positive lobe is limited by the desired resolution chosen by the FOV. The time that the gradient is left on, or the sampling time, is determined by the readout/receive bandwidth. If this time is doubled by the application of positive and negative lobes of the same amplitude and sampling, time is wasted within the pulse sequence. This wasted time results in less slices or, in the case of fast spin echo or EPI, shorter turbo factors and/or less slices. However, since it is the area under the lobes that must be equal, the negative lobe can have a higher amplitude and shorter sampling time and still complete the same area. This asymmetric gradient paradigm permits time savings in the sequence and hence more slices and/or longer turbo factors can be used (Fig. 12.4).

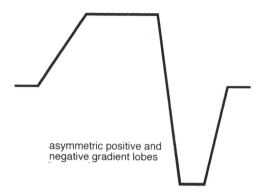

asymmetric positive and negative gradient lobes

Fig. 12.4 Asymmetric gradients.

Safety and power considerations

There are safety and power considerations associated with the application of high speed gradients. Rapid gradient switching can cause peripheral nerve stimulation. Such stimulation results in mild cutaneous sensations, muscle contractions and stimulation of the retinal phosphenes. For this reason, many ultra-fast gradient systems operate just below the stimulation threshold. The FDA limits gradient strength to 6 T/s for all gradients but permits 20T/s for axial gradients.

High speed gradient switching has high power requirements in the order of 1000 kW. This necessitates high quality gradient amplifiers. Resonant gradient systems, that oscillate at a particular frequency, provide a suitable alternative. Such systems produce a sinusoidal readout gradient which reduces gradient demands but are often incompatible with other imaging techniques that benefit from gradient switching (see Chapter 5).

Sampling sequelae

MR signals are sampled during readout when the frequency encoding gradient is applied. Signals are sampled only after the gradient has reached maximum amplitude. This type of sampling is known as conventional sampling. Unfortunately time is wasted within the pulse sequence waiting for the frequency encoding gradient to change.

Time within the sequence is reduced if sampling is performed while the frequency encoding gradient is changing. This is accomplished with a technique known as *ramp sampling* in which data points are collected when the rise time is almost complete. Sampling occurs while the gradient is still reaching maximum amplitude, while the gradient is at maximum amplitude and as is it begins to decline. However, this technique requires reconstruction programmes to reduce artefact and resolution may be lost (Fig. 12.5). Resonant gradient systems, that oscillate at a particular frequency, produce a sinusoidal readout gradient thereby permitting sinusoidal sampling. This technique provides an

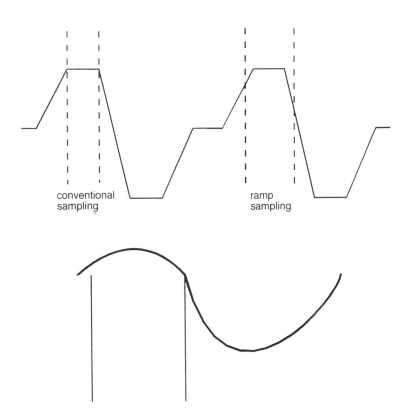

Fig. 12.5 A comparison between conventional and ramped sampling.

conventional sampling

ramp sampling

Fig. 12.6 Sinusoidal sampling.

efficient sampling mechanism but is not compatible with all imaging sequences (Fig. 12.6).

All of the previously described timesavings within pulse sequences can be translated into practical applications for MR system users. Such savings result in shorter imaging times, more slices and higher resolution matrices than in conventional imaging (Fig. 12.7). Practical developments of the new technology are now discussed.

Developments in fast spin echo

Fast spin echo pulse sequences save valuable imaging time by acquiring data information for several lines of K space per TR (see Chapter 5). The number of lines is determined by the turbo factor. The assignment of each line within K space is determined by the amplitude of the phase encoding gradient applied to each echo. High amplitude gradients encode information to the outer lines of K space and low amplitude gradients encode information for the centre of K space (see Fig. 5.6). In fast spin echo, image contrast is controlled by the TR and effective TE. The TR determines T1 contrast while the TE determines T2 contrast (Fig. 12.8). Since the centre of K space is responsible for contrast, the effective TE is the echo that is encoded for the centre of K space.

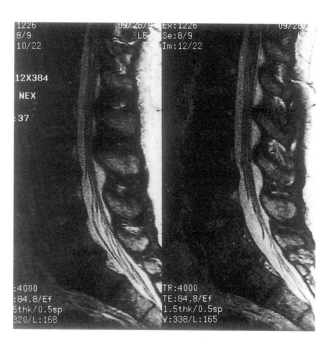

Fig. 12.7 These sagittal images of the spine were acquired using 2D fast spin echo with high speed gradient capabilities. Both images were acquired with similar imaging parameters and 1.5 mm slice thickness and 0 mm interslice gap. The image on the right was acquired with a 256 × 256 matrix whereas the image on the left was acquired with a 512 × 384 matrix. Note the exquisite resolution within the spinal canal.

As fast spin echo provides high quality images in shorter imaging times it has been utilised for a number of years as a suitable alternative for conventional T2 weighted spin echo acquisitions. Unfortunately fast spin echo imaging is not cost free. There are several trade-offs including image blurring and high signal from fat. As the infamous blurring is generally observed on long TR/short TE proton density weighted images, some centres continue to use conventional spin echo for this weighting. Alternatively shorter turbo factors minimise the artefact. High signal from fat can be easily remedied with fat suppression techniques such as spectral saturation. Studies have shown that fast spin echo with fat saturation techniques yield significantly higher contrast to noise than either gradient echo echo planar imaging (GE EPI) or spin echo echo planar imaging (SE EPI).

Single shot fast spin echo

It is now possible to acquire fast spin echo images in even shorter scan times by using a technique known as *single shot fast spin echo (SSFSE)*. In this technique all of the lines of K space are acquired in one TR. SSFSE combines a partial Fourier technique with fast spin echo. Half of the lines of K space are acquired in one TR and the other half are transposed (Fig. 12.9). This technique yields a reduction in imaging time as all of the image data is acquired in one TR, however there is a SNR penalty (Fig. 12.10).

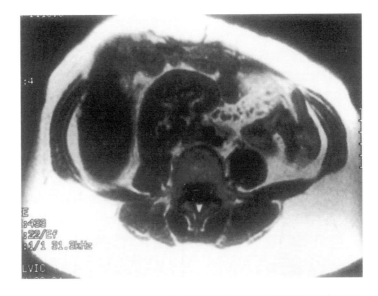

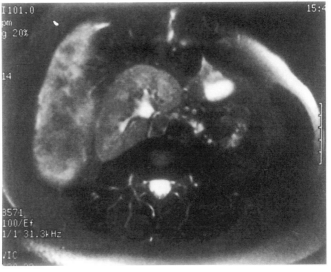

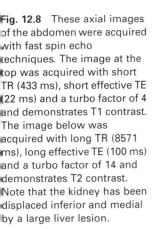

Fig. 12.8 These axial images of the abdomen were acquired with fast spin echo techniques. The image at the top was acquired with short TR (433 ms), short effective TE (22 ms) and a turbo factor of 4 and demonstrates T1 contrast. The image below was acquired with long TR (8571 ms), long effective TE (100 ms) and a turbo factor of 14 and demonstrates T2 contrast. Note that the kidney has been displaced inferior and medial by a large liver lesion.

3D fast spin echo

Even with high speed gradients, slice thickness is limited to 1 mm on most imaging systems. 3D fast spin echo acquisitions provide higher resolution and less susceptibility artefact than conventional gradient echo 3D acquisitions. 3D fast spin echo acquistions are acquired by the excitation of a slab (as opposed to a single slice), phase encoded (multiple lines of K space per TR period) and frequency encoded.

One of the main applications of 3D fast spin echo is the acquisition of high resolution T2 weighted images (Fig. 12.11). 3D fast spin echo has also proven useful for single breath-hold whole volume acquisitions of the

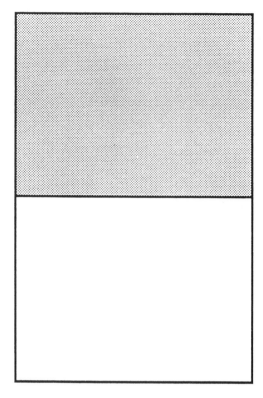

half K space
sampled in one
TR period

half K space
interpolated

Fig. 12.9 K space filling in
single shot fast spin echo.

Fig. 12.10 This axial image of
the abdomen was acquired
with a SSFSE technique. It was
acquired with long TR
(62 491 ms), long effective TE
(189 ms) for T2 information.
Compare this with Fig. 12.8
(T1 fast spin echo top and T2
fast spin echo bottom)
acquired from the same
patient at the same location.
Although the contrast is
similar to that of the image on
the right, the SNR is
compromised.

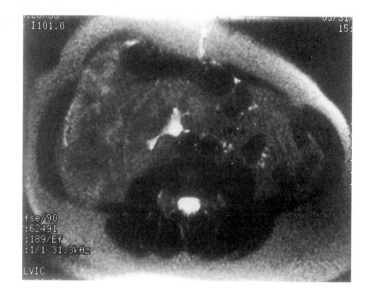

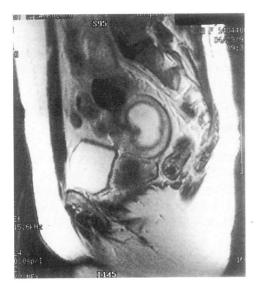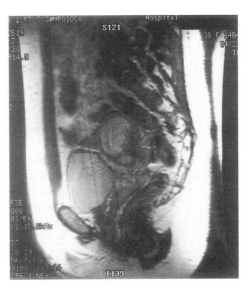

Fig. 12.11 These sagittal images of the pelvis were acquired with fast spin echo techniques. The image on the left was acquired with a 2D acquisition whereas the image on the right was acquired with a 3D acquisition. Although both have similar image contrast, the SNR on the 2D acquisition is superior to the 3D. However, the resolution on the 3D is superior despite the artefacts. This study was performed to rule out an ectopic pregnancy. Note that the fluid filled sac and the fetus is within the uterus.

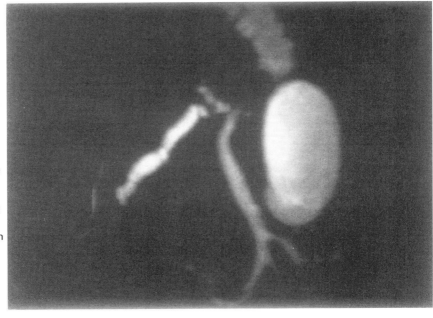

Fig. 12.12 This MRCP image was acquired using a 3D fast spin echo sequence. A very long TE (200 ms) and long TR (10 s) produces a heavily T2 weighted image where fluid in the biliary and pancreatic systems have a high signal intensity, and background tissues, with short T1 and T2 times, are suppressed.

liver and for MR cholangiopancreatography (MRCP) to evaluate duct conspicuity (Fig. 12.12). In addition, as cervical spine imaging requires high resolution and fast spin echo provides excellent myelographic effects, 3D fast spin echo is an excellent sequence choice in this area without the susceptibility effects found in 3D gradient echo acquisitions.

Developments in inversion recovery

In conventional spin echo inversion recovery sequences the modification of TI changes image contrast. For example, inversion recovery sequences with a short TI time (approximately 120–160 ms) suppress signal from fat (STIR). Inversion recovery sequences acquired with a long TI time suppress signal from CSF (FLAIR) (see Chapter 5) (Fig. 12.13).

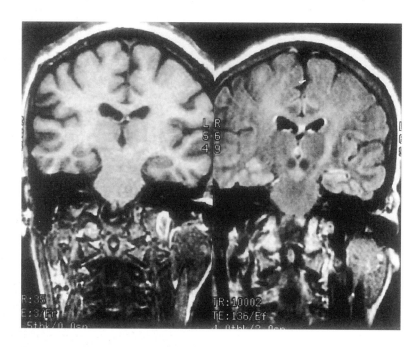

Fig. 12.13 Although at first glance they look similar, these coronal images of the brain were acquired for different information. The image on the left was acquired with a T1 spoiled or incoherent gradient echo for T1 information. The image on the right was acquired with a fast FLAIR acquisition for proton density information, but with dark signal from CSF. Note on the T1 gradient echo image the white matter is of higher signal intensity than the grey matter, whereas on the FLAIR image the grey matter is brighter than the white matter.

Inversion recovery sequences are generally acquired with a long TR and short TE and therefore result in long imaging times and produce few slice locations. During the TI waiting period prior to the excitation pulse, time is wasted within the imaging sequence. In fast inversion recovery acquisitions this time can be used to acquire additional slices. In addition, inversion recovery prep pulses can be added to fast spin echo or gradient echo acquisitions.

Spectral inversion recovery

The result of a marriage between fat saturation and STIR is an offspring known as spectral inversion recovery. In this a frequency selective, 180°

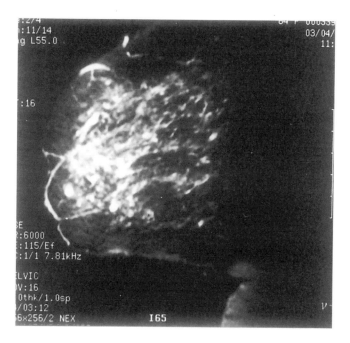

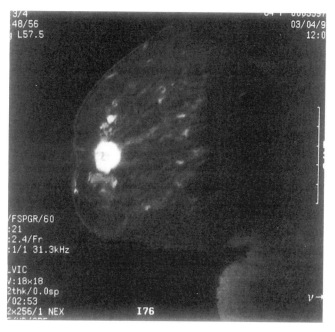

Fig. 12.14 These sagittal images of the breast were acquired to evaluate a suspected breast carcinoma. The image at the top was acquired with long TR (6000 ms) and long TE (115 ms) for T2 information. The image below was acquired with spectral inversion recovery applied to a fast T1 gradient echo after contrast enhancement. Note that the lesion is obscured on the T2 fast spin echo image by high signal from fluid within the ducts, whereas the lesion conspicuity is clearly better on the enhanced T1 fast gradient echo image with spectral saturation.

inversion recovery prep pulse is applied to the tissue prior to the scan. Spectral inversion recovery provides the uniform suppression of STIR and can also be used after contrast enhancement (Fig. 12.14).

Developments in gradient echo

Gradient echo pulse sequences use additional gradient pulses rather than RF pulses to refocus echoes. As gradient pulses are less time intensive than RF pulses, they permit shorter TRs and hence shorter imaging times. Contrast is maintained in short TR gradient echo sequences by modifying the flip angle. As the flip angle is shortened, less saturation occurs and less T1 contrast is present (see Chapter 1).

Unfortunately gradient echo sequences have several trade-offs. Since a RF refocusing pulse is not utilised, artefacts such as susceptibility and chemical shift commonly occur. However, these effects can be minimised or, in some cases, used to the advantage of the operator. For example, susceptibility effects are minimised by using short TEs as they allow less time for dephasing to occur. In addition, susceptibility may be further reduced by using small voxels which yield less intra-voxel dephasing and hence less artefact.

In some cases susceptibility artefacts help to differentiate lesions. Lesions which contain blood usually produce high susceptibility artefacts as blood products contain iron. Therefore susceptibility effects can be exploited with longer TEs and larger voxels, to improve visualisation of the lesion (Fig. 12.15).

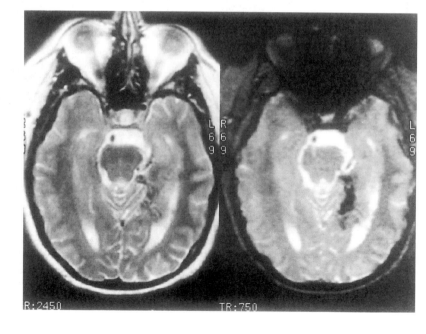

Fig. 12.15 These axial images of the brain were acquired to evaluate the arterio-venous malformation (AVM) in the posterior parietal lobe of the brain. The T2 fast spin echo (left) demonstrates subtle findings whereas the T2* gradient echo (right) shows a large susceptibility artefact in the same area caused by blood.

Fast gradient echo

Faster versions of the conventional gradient echo sequence have been developed which offer even shorter scan times. Fast gradient systems permit multi-slice gradient echo sequences with TEs as short as 0.7 ms. Multiple images can therefore be acquired in a single breath hold and are free from respiratory motion artefacts. In addition, fast gradient echo acquisitions are useful when temporal resolution is required. This is especially important after the administration of contrast when the selection of fast gradient echo permits dynamic imaging of an enhancing lesion. This important technique has applications in many areas including the abdominal viscera and the breast (Fig. 12.16).

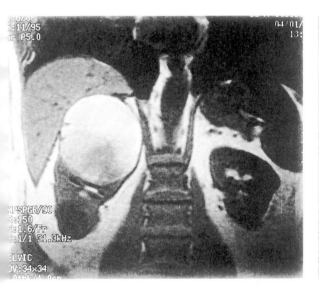

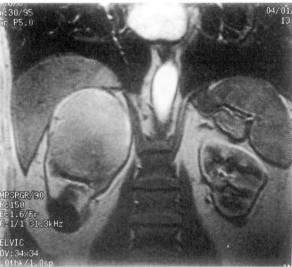

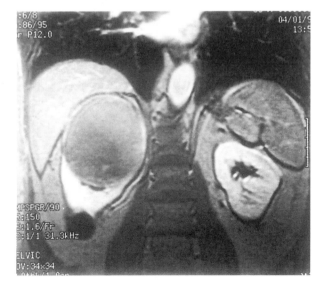

Fig. 12.16 These coronal images of the abdomen were acquired dynamically with an incoherent fast gradient echo acquisition for T1 information, during contrast enhancement. The first image (top left) was acquired before contrast was administered, the second (top right) was acquired 14 s into the injection and the last (bottom) was acquired 1 min after the injection had begun. Note the enhancement characteristics before, during, and almost after the injection was given. The lesion on the upper pole of the right kidney enhances whereas the renal cyst on the lower pole does not.

Fast 3D gradient echo imaging

Fast gradient echo images can be acquired in a 2D or 3D mode. For higher resolution images in rapid imaging times, a 3D fast gradient echo is optimal. This technique provides a high resolution dynamic image when acquired after contrast enhancement.

Applications of echo planar imaging (EPI)

EPI obtains images faster than any other mainstream imaging method by acquiring several lines of K space in one TR (see Chapter 5). EPI sequences can be configured in several different ways. Firstly, either a train of gradient echoes (GE EPI) or spin echoes (SE EPI) can be acquired.

Gradient echo EPI (GE EPI)

GE EPI is acquired with a RF pulse followed by a number of gradient blips creating a train of gradient echoes (see Fig. 5.34). In this scenario, images are acquired in one TR pass in milliseconds. Since gradient echoes are less time intensive than spin echoes, GE EPI can be acquired faster than SE EPI. Unfortunately GE EPI images demonstrate the same detrimental artefacts that are found in conventional gradient echo images.

Spin echo EPI (SE EPI)

To avoid some of the artefacts that are demonstrated with GE EPI, a RF refocusing pulse can be applied after the initial excitation pulse (see Fig. 5.33). The application of this refocusing pulse helps to clean up some of the artefacts caused by magnetic field inhomogeneities and chemical shift.

In addition to a selection between gradient echo and spin echo, the operator may also choose the type of data acquisition required. There are basically two alternatives: single shot and multi-shot.

Single shot EPI

Single shot EPI allows for all of the lines of K space to be acquired in one TR. This technique yields a significant reduction in imaging time as all of the image data is acquired in one TR pass, however there is a SNR and resolution penalty for this technique. To acquire EPI images with an acceptable level of artefact, the time between echoes must be minimised. For this reason, high speed gradients are required.

Multi-shot EPI

Multi-shot EPI images are acquired in several TR passes. In multi-shot EPI the effective time between echoes is dramatically reduced. As chemical shift, distortion and blurring are all proportional to echo spacing, artefacts in multi-shot EPI are reduced relative to single shot EPI.

Artefacts seen in EPI

Artefacts seen in EPI include those of all gradient echo sequences including distortion and chemical shift. Distortion is caused by magnetic field inhomogeneities. Since the magnetic field is not uniform, neither is the precessional frequency or phase. As a result frequency offsets cause a shift in the image but since the frequency is not uniform, the shift is not constant and geometric image distortion results especially in areas near air/water interfaces.

As each echo is acquired rapidly, chemical shift in the frequency direction is relatively small. However, as the sampling in the phase direction is similar to a slow narrow readout bandwidth, there is a larger chemical shift along the phase axis. This phase directional chemical shift artefact does not appear in standard spin or gradient echo acquisitions since echoes with different phase encodes are acquired at exactly the same time after excitation. The length of time required to acquire a train of phase encodes results in a small effective bandwidth of phase encode. For this reason in EPI, chemical shifts for fat are typically 10–20 pixels compared to the 1–2 pixel misregistration in spin echo imaging.

Other artefacts seen on EPI include blurring and ghosting. Blurring occurs as the result of $T2^*$ decay during the course of the EPI acquisition. If the train of echoes takes a similar time to decay, the signal from the end of the acquisition is reduced resulting in a loss of resolution and blurring. Half FOV ghosts occur as the result of small errors in the timing and shape of readout gradients. This causes differences between echoes acquired with positive and negative readout gradients. These errors cause a ghost of the real image that appears shifted in the phase direction by one half of the FOV. Since it is difficult to eliminate these errors, a correction is usually performed during image reconstruction using information acquired during the reference scan.

Body applications for EPI

Due to its high speed acquisition, the main applications of EPI are in the evaluation of structures that are in motion and where temporal resolution is paramount. In the body two such areas include the heart and the gastrointestinal tract. Studies are in progress to evaluate the clinical utility of ultra-fast, real-time MRI for the evaluation of gastrointestinal tract motility and cardiac function. The speed of EPI enables acquisition of

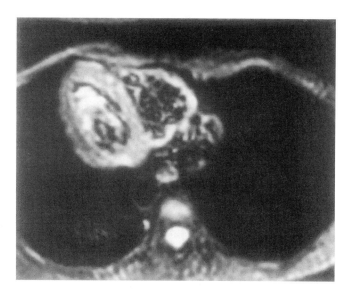

Fig. 12.17 This axial image of the heart was acquired with single shot EPI. Although the resolution of the image is marginal, this image was acquired in 20 ms.

images of the heart without the need for cardiac gating (Fig. 12.17). In addition, calculation of global cardiac function parameters can be validated using fast segmented K space, breath-hold, GE EPI images. In the gastrointestinal tract, peristaltic patterns of the gastric antrum and proximal small intestine can be depicted.

Neuro applications for EPI

EPI has many applications in the brain. EPI acquisitions can be used to acquire T2 and T2* weighted single slice images in milliseconds so that the entire brain can be imaged in as little as 2–3 s. In addition ultra-fast EPI sequences have permitted the evaluation of cerebral physiology and function using MRI. These techniques are now discussed in more detail.

Diffusion imaging

Diffusion is a term used to describe the movement of molecules due to random thermal motion. This motion is restricted by boundaries such as ligaments, membranes and macromolecules (Fig. 12.18). Sometimes restrictions in diffusion are directional, depending on the structure of the tissues. In early stroke, soon after the onset of ischaemia but before infarct or permanent tissue damage, cells swell and absorb water from the extracellular space. Since cells are full of large molecules and membranes, diffusion is restricted and the average diffusion in the tissue is reduced.

Spin echo imaging is, to a certain extent, structured to look at diffusion patterns in tissues. In spin echo acquisitions, spins with different frequencies are refocused (assuming they stay in the same place during excitation and refocusing). However, if spins move refocusing is not

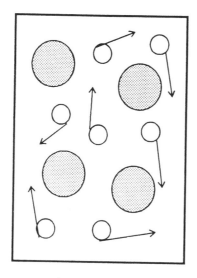 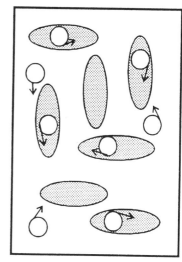

Fig. 12.18 Free and restricted diffusion of water.

freely diffusing water   restricted water

complete, and if motion is random signals cancel. If motion varies rapidly diffusion attenuation occurs and signal is lost in that area.

Diffusion weighted images can be more effectively acquired by combining EPI with two large gradient pulses applied after excitation. The gradient pulses are designed to cancel each other out if spins do not move, whilst moving spins experience phase shift. Therefore in diffusion imaging, signal attenuation occurs in normal tissues with random motion, and high signal appears in tissues with restricted diffusion (such as early stroke). The amount of attenuation depends on the amplitude and (possibly) the direction of the applied diffusion gradients.

Gradient pulses can be applied along the X, Y, and Z directions. Diffusion directions in the X, Y and Z axes are combined to produce a diffusion weighted image. When the diffusion gradients are applied only along the Y direction, or in the X direction, slight signal changes may reflect direction of axons. Diffusion gradients must be very long and very strong to achieve enough diffusion weighting. Diffusion sensitivity is controlled by a parameter 'b'. 'b' determines the diffusion attenuation by modification of the duration and amplitude of the diffusion gradient. 'b' can be expressed in units of s/mm^2. Typical 'b' values range from $500\,s/mm^2$, to $1000\,s/mm^2$.

As diffusion MRI uses a gradient system similar to phase contrast MRA, it is extremely prone to motion artefacts caused by phase changes. Even slight motion from cardiac pulsations and respiration cause phase changes. If a multi-shot sequence is used for diffusion imaging, phase changes will be different for different lines of K space and strong artefacts will appear along the phase direction. For this reason, diffusion weighted MR images are generally acquired with an ultra-fast technique such as SE EPI in conjunction with strong gradients. Additional echoes, known as navigator echoes, can be generated and then used to correct artefacts during post-processing.

Clinical applications for diffusion imaging are presently directed to the diagnosis of stroke. Early ischaemic lesions demonstrated by diffusion MRI represent regions with slower water diffusions due to intracellular water accumulation and/or shrinkage of the extracellular spaces (Fig. 12.19). Diffusion MRI can show not only irreversible but also reversible ischaemic lesions, and therefore has a potential to discriminate salvageable tissues from irreversibly damaged tissues before a therapeutic intervention. However, timing of diffusion MRI is important as it can only visualise fresh lesions as water diffusion is decreased several days after stroke onset.

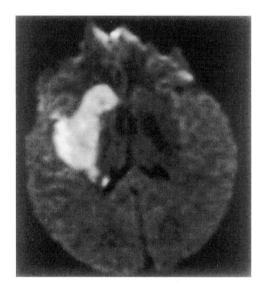

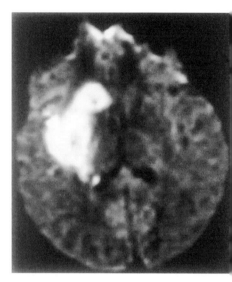

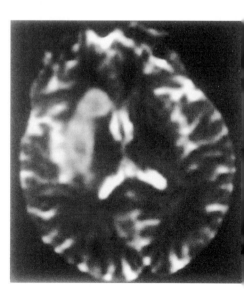

Fig. 12.19 Axial diffusion-weighted images of the brain acquired with a single shot EPI sequence and using different diffusion weighted gradients. The high signal intensity represents an area of infarct and restricted diffusion.

Perfusion imaging

Clinical perfusion measurements can be made with radio-tracers, but as MRI is a non-ionising technique with high spatial and temporal resolution that can be co-registered with anatomic information, there is much interest in perfusion MRI studies. Perfusion is the regional blood flow in tissues and is defined as the volume of blood which flows into one gram of tissue. Perfusion is a measure of the quality of vascular supply to a tissue and, since vascular supply and metabolism are usually related, perfusion can also be used to measure tissue activity.

Perfusion is measured using MRI by tagging the water in arterial blood during image acquisition. Tagging can be achieved by either a bolus injection of exogenous contrast agent like gadolinium, or by saturating the protons in arterial blood with RF inversion or saturation pulses. As the difference between tagged and untagged images is so small, ultra-fast imaging methods are desirable for reducing artefact. In its simplest form, perfusion images can be acquired with fast scanning acquisitions before, during and after a bolus injection of intravenous contrast. In this case several ultra-fast incoherent gradient echoes are acquired during breath hold at the same slice location. Since gadolinium shortens T1 recovery, visceral structures with high perfusion appear bright on T1 weighted fast gradient echoes. This technique is useful for the evaluation of visceral structures such as the kidneys, liver and spleen (see Fig. 12.16). Note the wash-in effect of contrast in the liver, spleen and kidneys.

Another technique to evaluate perfusion utilises a bolus injection of gadolinium administered intravenously during ultra-fast T2 or T2* acquisitions. In this case the contrast agent causes transient decreases in T2 and T2* decay in and around the microvasculature perfused with contrast. After data acquisition, a signal decay curve can be used to ascertain blood volume, transient time and measurement of perfusion. This curve is known as a time intensity curve. Time intensity curves for multiple images acquired during and after injection are combined to generate a cerebral blood volume (CBV) map.

Perfusion imaging with arterial spin tagging is another perfusion technique. With continuous arterial spin labelling (CASL), arterial spins are attenuated by inversion or saturation pulses outside the FOV. An untagged image is also acquired as a reference image. In this technique the reference image is subtracted from the tagged image. Spin tagging is a non-invasive alternative to the introduction of exogenous contrast agents that is potentially quantitative.

These techniques can be used to evaluate ischaemic disease or metabolism at rest or during exercise. In addition, the malignancy of neoplasms can be reflected in increased tissue metabolism or perfusion. On the CBV map, areas of low perfusion appear dark (stroke) whereas areas of higher perfusion appear bright (malignancies). Such techniques, albeit still in their infancy, show great potential in the evaluation of tissue viability and metabolism of vascular organs such as the heart, visceral structures and the brain.

Functional imaging (fMRI)

Functional MR imaging (fMRI) is a rapid MR imaging technique that acquires images of the brain during activity or stimulus and at rest. The two sets of images are then subtracted demonstrating functional brain activity as the result of increased blood flow to the activated cortex. In the early days of this technique visualisation of blood flow was achieved using contrast agents. More recently, however, the use of blood as an internal contrast is more widely used.

The magnetic properties of blood are important in the understanding of this technique. Haemoglobin is a molecule that contains iron and transports oxygen in the vascular system as oxygen binds directly to iron. When oxygen is bound (oxyhaemoglobin), the magnetic properties of iron are largely suppressed but when oxygen is not bound (deoxyhaemoglobin) the molecule becomes more magnetic. Therefore oxyhaemoglobin is diamagnetic and deoxyhaemoglobin is paramagnetic. Paramagnetic deoxyhaemoglobin creates an inhomogeneous magnetic field in its immediate vicinity. This inhomogeneous magnetic field increases $T2^*$ decay and attenuates signal from regions containing deoxyhaemoglobin.

At rest, tissue uses a substantial fraction of the blood flowing through the capillaries so venous blood contains an almost equal mix of oxyhaemoglobin and deoxyhaemoglobin. During exercise, however, when metabolism is increased, more oxygen is needed and hence more is extracted from the capillaries. In muscle tissue the concentration of oxyhaemoglobin in the venous system can become very low. The brain, however, is very sensitive to low concentrations of oxyhaemoglobin and therefore the cerebral vascular system increases blood flow to the activated area. Blood oxygenation actually increases during brain activity and specific locations of the cerebral cortex are activated during specific tasks. For example, seeing activates the visual cortex, hearing the auditory cortex, finger tapping the motor cortex, etc. More sophisticated tasks, including maze paradigms and other thought provoking tasks, stimulate other brain cortices.

The most important physiological effect that produces MR signal intensity changes between stimulus and rest is called *blood oxygenation level dependent (BOLD)*. BOLD exploits differences in the magnetic susceptibility of oxyhaemoglobin and deoxyhaemoglobin as a result of increased cerebral blood flow and little or no increase in local oxygen consumption that occurs during stimulation. Because deoxyhaemoglobin is paramagnetic, vessels containing a significant amount of this molecule create local field inhomogeneities causing dephasing and therefore signal loss. During activity, blood flow to the cortex increases causing a drop in deoxyhaemoglobin which results in a decrease in dephasing and a corresponding increase in signal intensity. These effects are very short lived and therefore require extremely rapid sequences such as EPI or fast gradient echo. To exploit $T2^*$ effects, BOLD images are usually acquired with long TEs (40–70 ms) while the task is modulated on and off. The 'off' images are then subtracted from the 'on' images and a more sophisticated statistical analysis is performed. Regions that were activated above some threshold level are overlaid on anatomical images (Fig. 12.20). It is these regions that reflect brain activity. With EPI, images can be collected in a very short time and therefore in principle high temporal resolution is possible. However, the temporal resolution is limited by a blurred intrinsic haemodynamic response and a finite SNR.

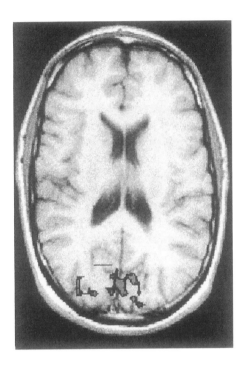

Fig. 12.20 This axial view of the brain was acquired for anatomical information. The irregular area overlaid on the posterior brain is the BOLD acquisition during visual stimulation. Note the increase in signal intensity resulting from increased activity in the visual cortex.

Despite these limitations there is no doubt that this sophisticated technique will develop our understanding of brain function and will have several clinical applications including the evaluation of stroke, epilepsy, pain and behavioural problems.

Interventional MRI

An exciting new development is the use of MRI for operative interventional procedures. The inherent safety and multi-planar facility of MRI makes it an ideal modality for some operative procedures. However, the development of this technique has required several modifications to existing hardware and software options.

Due to the restricted nature of conventional semi-conducting systems, a more open magnet design is required to permit easy access to the patient during the procedure. Low field permanent magnets are well suited from an access point of view, but image quality and acquisition times restrict their use to simple interventions. A new system utilises a semi-conducting

0.5 T system shaped liked two doughnuts which readily permits access to the patient and allows real-time image acquisition. This system permits intra-operative acquisition of MR images without moving the patient online image-guided stereotaxy without pre-operative imaging, and 'real-time' tracking of instruments in the operative field registered to the MR images. Precise location of the area under examination is achieved via triangulation and in-bore monitors permit continual monitoring of the procedure in three dimensions.

This is an expensive technique however. Flexible transmit and receive coils have been especially designed to fit around the operative area whilst allowing access for intervention. Endovascular coils have been developed to allow real-time tracking within vessels. In addition, all surgical instruments must be non-ferromagnetic and produce minimum susceptibility artefact so that they do not obscure the operating field. Anaesthetic and monitoring equipment must also be MR safe.

Despite these design and safety implications, the potential of interventional MR in the future is astounding and includes:

- liver imaging and tumour ablation with colorisation imaging capabilities,
- breast imaging and benign lump excision (Fig. 12.21),
- orthopaedic and kinematic studies,
- congenital hip dislocation manipulation and correction,
- biopsies.

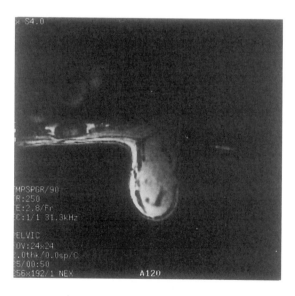

Fig. 12.21 Axial view of the breast acquired during MR guided needle aspiration of the suspicious ducts. In this case the lesion was only detected by MR and therefore could only be localised using MR.

One important application is tumour ablation using either laser therapy (in which heat is used to ablate the tumour) or cryotherapy (when extreme cold is used for ablation). MRI is the only imaging technique that can discriminate tissue of different temperatures. Since T1 recovery and T2 decay are temperature dependent, temperature changes alter image contrast. For this reason, techniques such as laser and cryotherapy can be monitored using MRI.

Interstitial laser therapy (ILT) is a promising therapeutic technique in which laser energy is delivered percutaneously to various depths in tissue. Previously the extent of heat distribution from the laser was difficult to assess. The use of EPI sequences has enabled real-time monitoring of laser-induced therapy providing a non-invasive method for intra-operative assessment of heat distribution during ILT. Similarly, interventional MR has enormous potential in the evaluation of cryotherapy.

This exciting new technique may have profound influences on interventional radiology. Although in its infancy, it is likely that in the future interventional vascular suites will be replaced by interventional MR systems and many surgical and interventional procedures will be carried out using MR technology.

Conclusion

It is evident that although we seem to have come a long way since the early days of MR, (remember the 20 min T2 spin echo sequence!), there is still an awfully long way to go. The potential applications of MRI are probably infinite. Although in this edition this chapter is called *Advanced Imaging Techniques*, in years to come the topics covered will almost certainly be considered routine. Watch this space!

Questions

1. High speed gradients provide a means for:
   (a) rapid imaging
   (b) high resolution imaging
   (c) functional imaging
   (d) all of the above.

2. The duty cycle is the:
   (a) percentage of time a gradient is permitted to work
   (b) oscillation of the B_1 field
   (c) strength of the gradient
   (d) rise time of the gradient.

3. SSFSE is a fast spin echo acquisition that:
   (a) fills multiple lines of K space in one TR
   (b) is acquired in one TR period
   (c) can fill half of K space and transpose the other half
   (d) all of the above.

4. Complete the sentence. ... images are generally acquired with contrast enhancement for dynamic imaging of the visceral structures.
   (a) Fast spin echo
   (b) Fast gradient echo
   (c) Fast IR
   (d) EPI.

5. Complete the sentence. ... images are acquired to diagnose stroke soon after onset of symptoms.
   (a) T1 weighted
   (b) T2 weighted
   (c) Proton density weighted
   (d) Diffusion weighted.

6. Deoxyhaemoglobin is:
   (a) paramagnetic
   (b) super-paramagnetic
   (c) diamagnetic
   (d) ferromagnetic.

7. fMRI utilises a technique known as:
   (a) FLAIR
   (b) BOLD
   (c) STIR
   (d) SSFSE.

8. MR can be used to monitor interventional procedures with a technique known as:
   (a) real-time
   (b) fluoro
   (c) quasi real-time
   (d) cine.

Glossary

Actual TE   the time between the echo and the next RF pulse in SSFP.

Aliasing   artefact produced when anatomy outside the FOV is mis-mapped inside the FOV.

Alnico   alloy that is used to make permanent magnets.

Angular momentum   the spin of MR active nuclei which depends on the balance between the number of protons and neutrons in the nucleus.

Atomic number   sum of protons in the nucleus.

B_0 the main magnetic field measured in Tesla.

Black blood imaging   acquisitions in which blood vessels are black.

Blood oxygen level dependent (BOLD)   a functional MRI technique that utilises the differences in magnetic susceptibility between oxyhaemoglobin and deoxyhaemoglobin to image of areas of activated cerebral cortex.

Bright blood imaging   acquisitions in which blood vessels are bright.

Central lines   area of K space filled with the shallowest phase encoding slopes.

Chemical misregistration   artefact along the phase axis caused by the phase difference between fat and water.

Chemical shift   artefact along the frequency axis caused by the frequency difference between fat and water.

Co-current flow   flow in the same direction as slice excitation.

Contrast to noise ratio CNR   difference in SNR between two points.

Counter current flow   flow in the opposite direction to slice excitation.

Cross excitation   energy given to nuclei in adjacent slices by the RF pulse.

Cross talk   energy given to nuclei in adjacent slices due to spin lattice relaxation.

Cryogens   substances used to super cool the coils of wire in a superconducting magnet.

Cryogen bath   area around the coils of wire in which cryogens are placed.

Decay   loss of transverse magnetisation.

Echo train   series of 180° rephasing pulse and echoes in a fast spin echo pulse sequence.

Effective TE   the time between the echo and the RF pulse that initiated it in SSFP.

Entry slice phenomena contrast difference of flowing nuclei relative to the stationary nuclei because they are fresh.

Even echo rephasing the use of evenly spaced echoes to reduce artefact.

Excitation the energy transfer from the RF pulse to the NMV.

Fast Fourier transform (FFT) mathematical conversion of frequency/time domain to frequency/amplitude.

Field of view (FOV) area of anatomy covered in an image.

Flip angle the angle of the NMV to B_0.

Flow encoding axes axes along which bipolar gradients act in order to sensitise flow along the axis of the gradient; used in phase contrast MRA.

Flow phenomena artefacts produced by flowing nuclei.

Flow related enhancement decrease in time of flight due to a decrease in velocity of flow.

Free induction decay (FID) loss of signal due to relaxation.

Frequency encoding locating a signal according to its frequency.

Fresh spins nuclei that have not been beaten down by repeated RF pulses.

Fringe field stray magnetic field outside the bore of the magnet.

Ghosting motion artefact in the phase axis.

Gibbs artefact line of low signal in the cervical cord due to truncation.

Gradient amplifier supplies power to the gradient coils.

Gradient echo echo produced as a result of gradient rephasing.

Gradient echo pulse sequence one that uses a gradient to regenerate an echo.

Gradients coils of wire that alter the magnetic field strength in a linear fashion when a current is passed through them.

Gradient spoiling the use of gradients to dephase magnetic moments. The opposite of rewinding.

Gyro-magnetic ratio the precessional frequency of an element at 1.0 T.

High velocity signal loss increase in time of flight due to an increase in the velocity of flow.

Homogeneity the evenness of the magnetic field.

Hybrid sequences combination of fast spin echo and EPI sequences where a series of gradient echoes are interspersed with spin echoes. In this way susceptibility artefacts are reduced.

In-flow effect another term for entry slice phenomenon.

Inhomogeneities areas where the magnetic field strength is not exactly the same as the main field strength – magnetic field unevenness.

Interleaving a method of acquiring data from alternate slices and dividing the sequence into two acquisitions; no slice gap is required.

Intra-voxel dephasing phase difference between flow and stationary nuclei in a voxel.

Ions atoms with an excess or deficit of electrons.

K space an area where data is stored.

Longitudinal plane the axis parallel to B_0.

Magnetic field gradient field created by passing current through a gradient coil.

Magnetic haemodynamic effect effect that causes elevation of the T wave of the ECG of the patient when placed in a magnetic field; this is due to the conductivity of blood.

Magnetic isocentre the centre of the bore of the magnet in all planes.

Magnetic moment denotes the direction of the north/south axis of a magnet and the amplitude of the magnetic field.

Magnetic susceptibility ability of a substance to become magnetised.

Magnetism a property of all matter that depends on the magnetic susceptibility of the atom.

Magnitude image unsubtracted image combination of flow sensitised data.

Mass number sum of neutrons and protons in the nucleus.

Maximum intensity projection technique that uses a ray passed through an imaging volume to assigned signal intensity according to their proximity to the observer.

MR active nuclei that possess an odd mass number.

MR angiography method of visualising vessels that contain flowing nuclei by producing a contrast between them and the stationary nuclei.

MR signal the voltage induced in the receiver coil.

Multiple overlapping thin section angiography (MOTSA) method combining a number of high resolution 3D acquisitions to produce an image that has good resolution and a large area of coverage.

Net magnetisation vector (NMV) the magnetic vector produced as a result of the alignment of excess hydrogen nuclei with B_0.

Number of signal averages the number of times an echo is encoded with the same slope of phase encoding gradient.

Nyquist theorem states that a frequency must be sampled at least twice in order to reproduce it reliably.

Ohms law basic law of electricity; $V = IR$.

Outer lines area of K space filled with the steepest phase encoding gradient slopes.

Partial averaging filling only a proportion of K space with data and putting zeros in the remainder.

Partial echo sampling only part of the echo and extrapolating the remainder in K space.

Partial saturation occurs when the NMV is flipped beyond 90° (91° to 179°).

Partial voluming loss of spatial resolution when large voxels are used.

Pathology weighting achieved in IR pulse sequence with a long TE; pathology appears bright even though the image is T1 weighted.

Permanent magnets magnets which retain their magnetism.

Phase the position of a magnetic moment on its precessional path at any given time.

Phase contrast angiography technique that generates vascular contrast by utilising the phase difference between stationary and flowing spins.

Phase encoding locating a signal according to its phase.

Phase image subtracted image combination of flow sensitised data.

Polarity the direction of a gradient, i.e. which end is greater than B_0 and which is lower than B_0. Depends on the direction of the current through the gradient coil.

Precession the secondary spin of magnetic moments around B_0.

Precessional (Larmor) frequency the speed of precession.

Proton density weighting image that demonstrates the differences in the proton densities of the tissues.

Pulse control unit co-ordinates the switching on and off of the gradient and RF transmitter coils at appropriate times during the pulse sequence.

Quenching process by which there is a sudden loss of the super conductivity of the magnet coils so that the magnet becomes resistive.

Ramp sampling where sampling data points are collected when the gradient rise time is almost complete. Sampling occurs while the gradient is still reaching maximum amplitude, while the gradient is at maximum amplitude and as it begins to decline.

Readout gradient the frequency encoding gradient.

Receive bandwidth range of frequencies that are sampled during readout.

Recovery growth of longitudinal magnetisation.

Relaxation process by which the NMV loses energy.

Repetition time TR time between each excitation pulse.

Residual transverse magnetisation transverse magnetisation left over from previous RF pulses in steady state conditions.

Resistive magnet another term for solenoid magnet.

Rewinding the use of a gradient to rephase magnetic moments.

RF amplifier supplies power to the RF transmitter coils.

RF pulse short burst of RF energy which excites nuclei into a high energy stage.

RF spoiling the use of digitised RF to transmit and receive at a certain phase.

RF transmitter coil   coil that transmits RF at the resonant frequency of hydrogen to excite nuclei and move them into a high energy state.

Rise time   the time it takes a gradient to switch on, achieve the required gradient slope, and switch off again.

RR interval   time between each R wave in gated studies.

Sampling rate   rate at which samples are taken during readout.

Sampling time   the time that the readout gradient is switched on for.

SAT TR   time between each pre-saturation pulse.

Saturation   occurs when the NMV is flipped to a full 180°.

Sequential acquisition   acquisition where all the data from each slice is acquired before going on to the next.

Shim coil   extra coils used to make the magnetic field as homogeneous as possible.

Shimming   process whereby the evenness of the magnetic field is optimised.

Signal to noise ratio SNR   ratio of signal relative to noise.

Single shot FSE (SSFSE)   a fast spin echo sequence where all the lines of K space are acquired during a single TR period.

Slice encoding   the separation of individual slice locations by phase in volume acquisitions.

Slice selection   selecting a slice using a gradient.

Solenoid electromagnet   magnet that uses current passed through coils of wire to generate a magnetic field.

Spatial modulation of magnetisation   creates a saturation effect which produces a cross hatching of stripes on the image; these can be compared with moving anatomy to determine its function.

Spatial resolution   the ability to distinguish two points as separate.

Spin down   the population of high energy hydrogen nuclei that align their magnetic moments anti-parallel to B_0.

Spin echo   echo produced as a result of a 180° rephasing pulse.

Spin echo pulse sequence   one that uses a 180° rephasing pulse to generate an echo.

Spin lattice relaxation   process by which energy is given up to the surrounding lattice.

Spin spin relaxation   process by which interactions between the magnetic fields of adjacent nuclei causes dephasing.

Spin up   the population of low energy hydrogen nuclei that align their magnetic moments parallel to B_0.

Superconducting magnet   solenoid electromagnet that uses super-cooled coils of wire so that there is no inherent resistance in the system; the current flows, and therefore the magnetism is generated without a driving voltage.

TAU   the time between the excitation pulse and the 180° rephasing pulse and the time between this and the echo.

3D volumetric acquisition   acquisition where the whole imaging volume is excited so that the images can be viewed in any plane.

Time of flight   rate of flow in a given time; causes some flowing nuclei to receive one RF pulse only and therefore produce a signal void.

Time of flight angiography   technique that generates vascular contrast by utilising the in-flow effect.

Time to echo TE   time between the excitation pulse and the echo.

T1 recovery   growth of longitudinal magnetisation as a result of spin lattice relaxation.

T1 time   time taken for 63% of the longitudinal magnetisation to recover.

T1 weighted image   image that demonstrates the differences in the T1 times of the tissues.

Transceiver   coil that both transmits RF and receives the MR signal.

Transmit bandwidth   range of frequencies transmitted in an RF pulse.

Transverse plane   the axis perpendicular to B_0.

Trigger delay   waiting period after each R wave; the time between the R wave and the beginning of data acquisition.

Trigger window   waiting period before each R wave in gated studies.

T2*   dephasing due to magnetic field inhomogeneities.

T2 decay   loss of transverse magnetisation as a result of spin spin relaxation.

T2 time   time taken for 63% of the transverse magnetisation to decay.

T2 weighted image   image that demonstrates the differences in the T2 times of the tissues.

Turbo factor or echo train length   the number of 180° rephasing pulse/echoes/phase encodings per TR in fast spin echo.

2D volumetric acquisition   acquisition where a small amount of data is acquired from each slice before repeating the TR.

Volume coil   coil that transmits and receives signal over a large volume of the patient.

Voxel volume   volume of tissue in the patient.

Window levels and settings   settings that control brightness and contrast in MR images.

UK versus US Spelling

Whilst compiling this book, we were aware that there are several words that are spelt differently in the UK and the US. We thought that it may be helpful to the reader to have a list of those words that came up regularly in the text.

UK	US
aluminium	aluminum
artefacts	artifacts
centre	center
colour	color
grey	gray
gynaecology	gynecology
haemorrhage	hemorrhage
haemostats	hemostats
initialisation	initialization
ischaemic	ischemic
magnetisation	magnetization
minimised	minimized
oedematous	edematous
orthopaedic	orthopedic

Further Reading

The following texts provide alternative and/or more in-depth discussions on many of the topics included in *MRI in Practice*.

Chapters 1–7

Bushong, S. (1996) *Magnetic Resonance Imaging: Physical and Biological Principles.* Moseby: St Louis, MO.

Cordoza, J. & Herfkens, R. (1994) *MRI Survival Guide.* Lippincott Raven: New York, NY.

English, P. & Moore, C. (1995) *MRI for Radiographers.* Springer Verlag: London.

Hashemi, R.H. & Bradley, W.G. Jr. (1997) *MRI: The Basics.* Williams and Wilkins: Baltimore: MD.

Kaut, C. (1992) *MRI Workbook for Technologists.* Lippincott Raven: New York, NY.

Kaut, C. & Faulkner, W. (1994) *Review Questions for MRI.* Blackwell Science: Oxford.

Ness Aiver, M. (1996) *All You Really Need to Know about MRI Physics.* University of Maryland: Baltimore.

Werhli, F. (1991) *Fast Scan Magnetic Resonance – Principles and Applications.* Raven Press: New York, NY.

Westbrook, C. (1994) *Handbook of MRI Technique.* Blackwell Science: Oxford.

Wheeler, G. & Withers, K. (1996) *Lippincott Magnetic Resonance Imaging Review.* Lippincott Raven: New York, NY.

Chapter 8

Adamis, M.K., Li, W., Wielopolski, P.A., Kim, D., Sax, E.J., Kent, K.C. & Edelman, R.R. (1995) Dynamic contrast-enhanced subtraction MR angiography of the lower extremities: initial evaluation with a multisection, two-dimensional time-of-flight sequence. *Radiology*, **196**(3), 689–95.

Cloft, H.J., Murphy, K.J., Prince, M.R. & Brunberg, J.A. (1996) D gadolinium-enhanced MR angiography of the carotid arteries. *Magnetic Resonance Imaging*, **14**(6), 593–600.

Colletti, P.M. & Terk M.R. (1996) Magnetic resonance imaging applications to cardiac diagnosis. *Biomedical Instrument Technology*, **30**(4), 354–8.

Cortell, E.D., Kaufman, J.A., Geller S.C., Cambria, R.P., Rivitz, S.M. & Waltman, A.C. (1996) MR angiography of tibial runoff vessels: imaging with the head coil compared with conventional arteriography. *American Journal of Roentgenology*, **167**(1), 147–51.

Fayad, Z.A., Connick, T.J. & Axel, L. (1995) An improved quadrature or phased-array coil for MR cardiac imaging. *Magnetic Resonance in Medicine*, **34**(2), 186–93.

Gai, N. & Axel, L. (1996) Correction of motion artifacts in linogram and projection reconstruction MRI using geometry and consistency constraints. *Medical Physics*, **23**(2), 251–62.

Gimbel, J.R., Johnson, D., Levine P.A. & Wilkoff, B.L. (1996) Safe performance of magnetic resonance imaging on five patients with permanent cardiac pacemakers. *Pacing and Clinical Electrophysiology*, **19**(6), 913–19.

Glickerman, D.J., Obregon, R.G., Schmiedl, U.P., Harrison, S.D., Macaulay, S.E., Simon, H.E. & Kohler, T.R. (1996) Cardiac-gated MR angiography of the entire lower extremity: a prospective comparison with conventional, angiography. *American Journal of Roentgenology*, **167**(2), 445–51.

Haacke, E.M., Li, D. & Kaushikkar, S. (1995) Cardiac MR imaging: principles and techniques. *Topics in Magnetic Resonance Imaging*, **7**(4), 200–17.

Hatabu, H., Gefter, W.B., Axel, L., Palevsky, H.I., Cope, C., Reichek, N., Doughterty, L., Listerud, J. & Kressel, H.Y. (1994) MR imaging with spatial modulation of magnetization in the evaluation of chronic central pulmonary thromboemboli. *Radiology*, **190**(3), 791–6.

Holland, G.A., Dougherty, L., Carpenter, J.P., Golden, M.A., Gilfeather, M., Slossman, F., Schnall, M.D. & Axel, L. (1996) Breath-hold ultrafast three-dimensional gadolinium-enhanced MR angiography of the aorta and the renal and other visceral abdominal arteries. *American Journal of Roentgeology*, **166**(4), 971–81.

Hundley, W.G., Li, H.F., Willard, J.E., Landau, C., Lange, R.A., Meshack, B.M., Hillis, L.D. & Peshock, R.M. (1995) Magnetic resonance imaging assessment of the severity of mitral regurgitation. Comparison with invasive techniques. *Circulation*, **92**(5), 1151–8.

Loubeyre, P., Trolliet, P. Cahen, R. Grozel, F., Labeeuw, M. & Minh, V.A. (1996) MR angiography of renal artery stenosis: value of the combination of three-dimensional time-of-flight and, three-dimensional phase-contrast MR angiography sequences. *American Journal of Roentgenology*, **167**(2), 489–94.

Stringaris, K., Liberopoulos K., Giaka E., Kokkinis, K., Bastounis, E., Klonaris, E.C. & Balas, P. (1996) Three-dimensional time-of-flight MR angiography and MR imaging versus conventional angiography in carotid artery dissections. *International Angiology*, **15**(1), 20–25.

Chapter 9

Claasen-Vujcic, T., Borsboom, H.M., Gaykema, H.J. & Mehlkopf, T. (1996) Transverse low-field RF coils in MRI. *Magnetic Resonance in Medicine*, **36**(1), 111–16.

Davis, C.P., McKinnon, G.C., Debatin, J.F. & von Schulthess, G.K. (1996) Ultra-high-speed MR imaging. *European Radiology*, 6(3), 297–311.

Fried, M.P., Hsu, L. Topulos, G.P. & Jolesz, F.A. (1996) Image-guided surgery in a new magnetic resonance suite: preclinical considerations. *Laryngoscope*, **106**(4), 411–17.

General Electric (1982) *NMR Site Planning Considerations.* General Electric Applications Guide number 5435A.

Maier, C.F., Chu, K.C., Chronik, B.A. & Rutt, B.K. (1995) A novel transverse gradient coil design for high-resolution MR imaging. *Magnetic Resonance in Medicine*, **34**(4), 604–11.

Mansfield, P., Chapman, B.L., Bowtell, R., Glover, P., Coxon, R., & Harvey P.R.

(1995) Active acoustic screening: reduction of noise in gradient coils by Lorentz force balancing. *Magnetic Resonance in Medicine*, **33**(2), 276–81.

Schnall, M.D., Connick, T., Hayes, C.E., Lenkinski, R.E. & Kressel, H.Y. (1992) MR imaging of the pelvis with an endo-rectal external multicoil array. *Journal of Magnetic Resonance Imaging*, **2**, 229–32.

Sorgenfrei, B.L. & Edelstein, W.A. (1996) Optimizing MRI signal-to-noise ratio for quadrature unmatched RF coils: two preamplifiers are better than one. *Magnetic Resonance in Medicine*, **36**(1), 104–10.

Wen, H., Jaffer, F.A., Denison, T.J., Duewell, S., Chesnick, A.S. & Balaban, R.S. (1996) The evaluation of dielectric resonators containing H_2O or D_2O as RF coils for high-field MR imaging and spectroscopy. *Journal of Magnetic Resonance Series B*, **110**(2), 117–23.

Chapter 10

Kanal, E. (1996) Echo-planar MR imaging [letter, comment]. *Radiology*, **198**(2), 585–6.

Kanal, E., Shellock, F.G. & Lewin, J.S. (1996) Aneurysm clip testing for ferromagnetic properties: clip variability issues. *Radiology*, **200**(2), 576–8.

Kanal, E. & Shaibani, A. (1994) Firearm safety in the MR imaging environment [comments]. *Radiology*, **193**(3), 875–6.

Kanal, E., Shellock, F.G. & Talagala, L. (1990) Safety considerations in MR imaging. *Radiology*, **176**(3), 593–606.

Shellock, F.G. (1986) Monitoring during MRI: an evaluation of the effect of high field MRI in various patient monitors. *Medical Electronics*, Sept, 93–7.

Shellock, F.G. (1991) MRI and implantable vascular access ports. *Journal of Magnetic Resonance Imaging*, **1**(2), 243.

Shellock, F.G. & Crues, J.V. (1988) Corneal temperature changes associated with high field strength MR imaging using a head coil. *Radiology*, **167**(3), 809–11.

Shellock, F.G. & Crues, J.V. (1988) Temperature changes caused by MR imaging of the brain with a head coil. *American Journal of Neuro-Radiology*, **9**(2), 287–91.

Shellock, F.G. & Kanal, E. (1991) SMRI Safety Committee. Policies, guidelines and recommendations for MR imaging safety and patient management. *Journal of Magnetic Resonance Imaging*, **1**(1), 97–101.

Shellock, F.G. & Kanal, E. (1994) Guidelines and recommendations for MR imaging safety and patient management. III. Questionnaire for screening patients before MR procedures. The SMRI Safety Committee. *Journal of Magnetic Resonance Imaging*, **4**(5), 749–51.

Shellock, F.G., Schaefer, D.J. & Crues, J.V. (1989) Alterations in body and skin temperatures caused by MRI: is the recommended exposure for radio-frequency radiation too conservative? *British Journal of Radiology*, **62**(742), 904–909.

Shellock, F.G., Schaefer, D.J. & Gordon, C.J. (1986) Effect of a 1.5 T static magnetic field on body temperature of man. *Magnetic Resonance in Medicine*, **3**, 644–7.

Shellock, F.G. & Schatz, C.J. (1991) Metallic otologic implants: in vitro assessments of ferromagnetism at 1.5 T. *American Journal of Neuro-Radiology*, **12**, 279–81.

Shellock, F.G. & Shellock, V.J. (1996) Vascular acces ports and catheters: ex vivo testing of ferromagnetism, heating, and artifacts associated with MR imaging. *Magnetic Resonance Imaging*, **14**(4), 443–7.

Chapter 11

Bloem, J.L., Reiser, M.F. & Vanel, D. (1990) Magnetic resonance contrast agents in the evaluation of the musculo-skeletal system. *Magnetic Resonance Quarterly*, **6**(2) 136–63.

Buxton, P.J. (1996) Short communication: the use of sodium ironedetate (Sytron) as an MRI rectal contrast agent. *British Journal of Radiology*, **69**(819), 266–8.

Chang, C.A., Sieving, P.F., Watson, A.D. & Dewey, T.M. (1992) Ionic versus non-ionic MR imaging contrast media: operational definitions. *Journal of Magnetic Resonance Imaging*, **2**(1), 95–8.

Engelstad, B.L. & Wolf, G.L. (1992) *Contrast Agents.* Chapter 9; 161–199.

Grangier, C., Tourniaire, J., Mentha, G., Schiau, R., Howarth, N., Chachuat, A., Grossholz, M. & Terrier, F. (1994) Enhancement of liver hemangiomas on T1-weighted MR SE images by superparamagnetic iron oxide particles. *Journal of Computer Assisted Tomography*, **18**(6), 888–96.

Imakita, S., Nishimura, T., Yamada, N. & Naito, H. (1988) Magnetic resonance imaging of cerebral infarction: time course of Gd-DTPA enhancement and CT comparison. *Neuroradiology*, **30** 372–8.

Johnson, W.K., Stoupis, C., Torres, G.M., Rosenberg, E.B. & Ros, P.R. (1996) Superparamagnetic iron oxide (SPIO) as an oral contrast agent in gastrointestinal (GI) magnetic resonance imaging (MRI): comparison with state-of-the-art computed tomography (CT). *Magnetic Resonance Imaging*, **14**(1), 43–9.

Krieg, F.M., Andres, R.Y. & Winterhalter, K.H. (1995) Superparamagnetically labelled neutrophils as potential abscess-specific contrast agent for MRI. *Magnetic Resonance Imaging*, **13**(3), 393–400.

Lin, W., Haacke, E.M., Smith, A.S. & Clampitt, M.E. (1992) Gadolinium enhanced high resolution MR angiography with adaptive vessel tracking: preliminary results in the intra-cranial circulation. *Journal of Magnetic Resonance Imaging*, **2**(3), 277–84.

Maravilla, K.R. (1991) Optimal use of MR contrast agents: how much is enough? *American Journal of Neuro-Radiology*, **12**, 881–3.

Mathur-De Vré, R. & Lemort, M. (1995) Invited review: biophysical properties and clinical applications of magnetic resonance imaging contrast agents. *British Journal of Radiology*, **68**(807), 225–47.

Reimer, P., Schuierer, G., Balzer, T. & Peters, P.E. (1995) Application of a superparamagnetic iron oxide (Resovist) for MR imaging of human cerebral blood volume. *Magnetic Resonance in Medicine*, **34**(5), 694–7.

Runge, V.M. & Wells, J.W. (1995) Update: safety, new applications, new MR agent. *Topics in Magnetic Resonance Imaging*, **7**(3) 181–95.

Sherry, A.D., Cacheris, W.P. & Kuan, K.T. (1988). Stability constants for Gd3+binding to model DTPA-conjugates and DTPA-proteins: implications for their use as magnetic resonance contrast agents. *Magnetic Resonance in Medicine*, 180–90.

Chapter 12

Alsop, D.C. (1997) The sensitivity of low flip angle RARE imaging. *Magnetic Resonance in Medicine*, **37**(2), 176–84.

Alsop, D.C. & Detre, J.A. (1996) Reduced transit-time sensitivity in noninvasive magnetic resonance imaging of human cerebral blood flow. *Journal of Cerebral Blood Flow and Metabolism*, **16**(6), 1236–49.

Alsop, D.C., Hatabu, H., Bonnet, M., Listerud, J. & Gefter, W. (1995) Multi-slice, breathhold imaging of the lung with submillisecond echo times. *Magnetic Resonance in Medicine*, **33**(5), 678–82.

Alsop, D.C., Murai, H., Detre, J.A., McIntosh, T.K. & Smith, D.H. (1996) Detection of acute pathologic changes following experimental traumatic brain injury using diffusion-weighted magnetic resonance imaging. *Journal of Neurotrauma*, **13**(9), 515–21.

Armstrong, F.D., Thompson, R.J. Jr, Wang, W., Zimmerman, R., Pegelow, C.H., Miller, S., Moser, F., Bello, J., Hurtig, A. & Vass, K. (1997) Cognitive functioning and brain magnetic resonance imaging in children with sickle cell disease. *Paediatrics*, **97** (6, Part 1), 864–70.

Baum, K.A., Schulte, C., Girke, W., Reischies, F.M. & Felix, R. (1996) Incidental white-matter foci on MRI in 'healthy' subjects: evidence of subtle cognitive dysfunction. *Neuroradiology*, **38**(8), 755–60.

Bloomgarden, D.C., Fayad, Z.A., Ferrari, V.A., Chin, B., Sutton, M.G. & Axel, L. (1997) Global cardiac function using fast breath-hold MRI: validation of new acquisition and analysis techniques. *Magnetic Resonance in Medicine*, **37**(5), 683–92.

Colletti, P.M. (1996) Computer-assisted imaging of the fetus with magnetic resonance imaging. *Computerised Medical Imaging and Graphics*, **20**(6), 491–6.

Crawley, A.P., Cohen, M.S., Yucel, E.K., Poncelet, B. & Brady, T.J. (1992) Single-shot magnetic resonance imaging: applications to angiography. *Cardiovascular Interventional Radiology*, **15**(1), 32–42.

Crnac, J., Schmidt, M.C., Theissen, P. & Sechtem, U. (1997) Assessment of myocardial perfusion by magnetic resonance imaging. *Herz*, **22**(1), 16–28.

Davis, C.P., McKinnon, G.C., Debatin, J.F. & von Schulthess, G.K. (1996) Ultra-high-speed MR imaging. *European Radiology*, **6**(3), 297–311.

Duyn, J.H., Yang, Y., Frank, J.A., Mattay, V.S. & Hou, L. (1996) Functional magnetic resonance neuroimaging data acquisition techniques. *Neuroimage*, **4**(3), S76–S83.

Eddy, W.F., Fitzgerald, M. & Noll, D.C. (1996) Improved image registration by using Fourier interpolation. *Magnetic Resonance in Medicine*, **36**(6), 923–31.

Georgy, B.A. & Hesselink, J.R. (1994) MR imaging of the spine: recent advances in pulse sequences and special techniques. *American Journal of Roentgenology*, **162**(4), 923–34.

Gilfeather, M., Holland, G.A., Siegelman, E.S., Schnall, M.D., Axel, L., Carpenter, J.P. & Golden, M.A. (1997) Gadolinium-enhanced ultrafast three-dimensional spoiled gradient-echo MR imaging of the abdominal aorta and visceral and iliac vessels. *Radiographics*, **17**(2), 423–32.

Gmitro, A.F., Ehsani, A.R., Berchem, T.A. & Snell, R.J. (1996) A real-time reconstruction system for magnetic resonance imaging. *Magnetic Resonance in Medicine*, **35**(5), 734–40.

Gudbjartsson, H., Maier, S.E., Mulkern, R.V., Morocz, I.A., Patz, S. & Jolesz, F.A. (1996) Line scan diffusion imaging. *Magnetic Resonance in Medicine*, **36**(4), 509–19.

Harada, J. (1997) Principle and clinical application of MRI. *Rinsho Byori*, **45**(3), 237–41.

Ichikawa, T., Nitatori, T., Hachiya, J. & Mizutani, Y. (1996) Breath-held MR cholangiopancreatography with half-averaged single shot hybrid rapid acquisition with relaxation enhancement sequence: comparison of fast GRE and SE sequences. *Journal of Computer Assisted Tomography*, **20**(5), 798–802.

Jara, H., Soto, J.A., Yu, B., Hentzen, P.C., van Yperen, G.H. & Yucel, E.K. (1996) Multisection T1-weighted hybrid-RARE: a pulse sequence for MR imaging of the entire liver during suspended respiration. *Magnetic Resonance in Medicine*, **36**(5), 767–74.

Jezzard, P. & Song, A.W. (1996) Technical foundations and pitfalls of clinical fMRI. *Neuroimage*, **4**(3), S63–S75.

Kim, S.G., Richter, W. & Ugurbil, K. (1997) Limitations of temporal resolution in functional MRI. *Magnetic Resonance in Medicine*, **37**(4), 631–6.

Kukkonen, C.A. (1995) NASA high performance computing, communications, image processing, and data visualization-potential applications to medicine. *Journal of Medical Systems*, **19**(3), 263–73.

Lee, C.C., Jack, C.R. Jr, Grimm, R.C., Rossman, P.J., Felmlee, J.P., Ehman, R.L. & Riederer, S.J. (1996) Real-time adaptive motion correction in functional MRI. *Magnetic Resonance in Medicine*, **36**(3), 436–44.

Lufkin, R. (1989) Approaches to fast MR imaging. *Computerised Medical Imaging and Graphics*, **13**(2), 145–51.

Ma, J., Wehrli, F.W. & Song, H.K. (1996) Fast 3D large-angle spin-echo imaging (3D FLASE). *Magnetic Resonance in Medicine*, **35**(6), 903–10.

Minematsu, K., Hasegawa, Y. & Yamaguchi, T. (1995) Diffusion MRI for evaluating cerebrovascular disease. *Rinsho Shinkeigaku*, **35**(12), 1575–7.

Moriarty, T. M., Kikinis, R., Jolesz, F.A., Black, P.M., & Alexander, E. (1996) Magnetic resonance imaging therapy. Intraoperative MR imaging. *Neurosurgical Clinics of North America*, **7**(2), 323–31.

Naganawa, S., Jenner, G., Cooper, T.G., Potchen, E.J. & Ishigaki, T. (1994) Rapid MR imaging of the liver: comparison of twelve techniques for single breath-hold whole volume acquisition. *Radiation Medicine*, **12**(6), 255–61.

Orel, S.G., Hochman, M.G., Schnall, M.D., Reynolds, C. & Sullivan, D.C. (1996) High-resolution MR imaging of the breast: clinical context. *Radiographics*, **16**(6), 1385–401.

Pushek, T., Farahani, K., Saxton, R.E., Soudant, J., Lufkin, R., Paiva, M. & Jongewaard, N. (1995) Dynamic MRI-guided interstitial laser therapy: a new technique for minimally invasive surgery. *Laryngoscope*, **105**(11), 1245–52.

Rehwald, W.G., Reeder, S.B., McVeigh, E.R. & Judd, R.M. (1997) Techniques for high-speed cardiac magnetic resonance imaging in rats and rabbits. *Magnetic Resonance in Medicine* **37**(1), 124–30.

Riederer, S.J. (1996) Recent technical advances in MR imaging of the abdomen. *Magnetic Resonance Imaging*, **6**(5), 822–32.

Roberts, T.P., Vexler, Z.S., Vexler, V., Derugin, N. & Kucharczyk, J. (1996) Sensitivity of high-speed 'perfusion-sensitive' magnetic resonance imaging to mild cerebral ischemia. *European Radiology*, **6**(5), 645–9.

Schenck, J.F. (1996) The role of magnetic susceptibility in magnetic resonance imaging: MRI magnetic compatibility of the first and second kinds. *Medical Physics*, **23**(6), 815–50.

Sebag, G., Pointe, H.D., Klein, I., Maiza, D., Mazda, K., Bensahel, H., & Hassan, M. (1997) Dynamic gadolinium-enhanced subtraction MR imaging – a simple technique for the early diagnosis of Legg-Calve-Perthes disease: preliminary results. *Pediatric Radiology*, **27**(3), 216–20.

Sinha, U. & Sinha, S. (1996) High speed diffusion imaging in the presence of eddy currents. *Journal of Magnetic Resonance Imaging*, **6**(4): 657–66.

Sorensen, A.G., Tievsky, A.L., Ostergaard, L., Weisskoff, R.M. & Rosen, B.R. (1997) Contrast agents in functional MR imaging. *Magnetic Resonance Imaging*, **7**(1), 47–55.

Stehling, M.K., Evans, D.F., Lamont, G., Ordidge, R.J., Howseman, A.M. Chapman, B. & Coxon, R. (1989) Gastrointestinal tract: dynamic MR studies with echo-planar imaging. *Radiology*, **171**(1): 41–6.

Steiner, P., McKinnon, G.C., Romanowski, B., Goehde, S.C., Hany, T., & Debatin, J.F. (1997) Contrast-enhanced, ultrafast 3D pulmonary MR angiography in a single breath-hold: initial assessment of imaging performance. *Magnetic Resonance Imaging*, **7**(1), 177–82.

Yang, Y., Mattay, V.S., Weinberger, D.R., Frank, J.A. & Duyn, J.H. (1997) Localized echo-volume imaging methods for functional MRI. *Magnetic Resonance Imaging*, **7**(2), 371–5.

Yoshikawa, K., Tobe, K., Yoshioka, N. & Yoshida, H. (1996) MR imaging and dynamic MR imaging. *Nippon Rinsho*, **54**(5), 1255–62.

Note: Most of the main manufacturers publish applications manuals some of which include the principles of physics. The manuals produced by GE and Philips are particularly good.

Answers to Questions

Chapter 1

1. The Larmor equation states that the resonant frequency is equal to the gyro-magnetic ratio multiplied by the main magnetic field strength. It calculates resonant frequency for a specific element at a specific field strength.
2. RF pulse perpendicular to B_0 and at the resonant frequency.
3. b
4. Transverse magnetisation that is in phase.
5. Time taken for 63% of the longitudinal magnetisation to recover.
6. Time for 63% of the transverse magnetisation to decay due to dephasing.
7. T1 recovery affects the angle of the NMV to the main magnetic field.
   T2 decay affects dephasing of magnetic moments in the NMV.
   Proton density affects the number of nuclei in the NMV.
8. (a) TR.
   (b) TE.

Chapter 2

1. T1, T2 and proton density contrast affects every image regardless of the pulse sequence and parameters. We can never acquire a purely T1 image. Therefore we select parameters to weight the image towards one process and away from the other two.
2. (a) A T1 weighted image is an image whose contrast is predominantly due to the differences in the T1 recovery times of the tissues.
   (b) A T2 weighted image is an image whose contrast is predominantly due to the differences in the T2 decay times of the tissues.
   (c) A proton density weighted image is an image whose contrast is predominantly due to the differences in the proton densities of the tissues.
3. a
4. The TR must be short so that neither fat nor water have had time to fully recover their longitudinal magnetisation. Fat will have recovered further than water and so T1 contrast will be maximised. The TE must also be short to minimise the T2 differences between the tissues.
5. A 180° pulse rephases the dephased magnetic moments caused by inhomogeneities in the field. This enables true T2 to be measured.
6. Variable flip angles, gradient rephasing, shorter TRs and scan times.
7. TR and the flip angle.
8. (a) T1 weighting.
   (b) T2* weighting.

Chapter 3

1. Slice selection, phase encoding, frequency encoding.
2. The direction of the current through the gradient coil.
3. The FOV.
4. The matrix.
5. K space is where data is stored in the array processor.
6. The Nyquist theorem states that data must be sampled at least twice per cycle in order to reproduce it accurately.
7. (a) The right-hand side of K space only is sampled. The left-hand side is extrapolated from the right-hand side. Shorter TEs are therefore allowed.
   (b) Only a proportion of the lines of K space are filled with data. The rest is filled with zeroes. The scan time and SNR are decreased as a result.

Chapter 4

1. The ability to resolve. The minimum distance between two points at which they can be seen as distinct and separate.
2. (a) 256×256, 3 mm slice thickness, 12 cm FOV, 1 NEX.
   (b) 512×256, 4 mm slice thickness, 8 cm FOV, 2 NEX.
3. MTC, T2 weighted images, contrast enhancement.
4. Use a surface coil to improve SNR.
   Reduce the TR to reduce the scan time.
   16 slices are not usually required in a cervical spine examination, 10 or 12 will suffice.
   Use rectangular FOV if available to increase resolution.
   NEX may be increased if necessary, but watch that the scan time is not too long for the patient to tolerate.
   Increase the FOV to 24 cm as this will increase the SNR fourfold.
   Increase the slice thickness slightly, e.g. 4 mm.
5. The incremental step between each phase encode is doubled which halves the FOV in the phase direction and halves the number of phase encodes performed. The resolution is maintained but the scan time is halved.
6. Volumes allow contiguous slices to be acquired.
   Thinner slices achievable (less than 1 mm).
   SNR increased because whole volume is being excited.
   Reformatting in any plane possible.
7. Voxel must be isotropic, i.e. equal dimensions in all planes.
   Keep matrix square.
   Calculate pixel dimension by dividing FOV by number of pixels.
   Select slice thickness that equals this dimension.

Chapter 5

1. (a) 2D incoherent gradient echo.
   (b) Coherent gradient echo.
   (c) SSFP.
2. RF spoiling eliminates residual transverse magnetisation that causes increased T2* weighting.

3. SSFP produces images with long TEs so T1 weighting is minimised.
4. Gradient echo sequences use a gradient to rephase, have variable flip angles, have faster scan times and more artefact than spin echo sequences.
5. Shorter scan times, more T2 weighting, less slices per TR.
6. In coherent gradient echo the FID and the spin echo are sampled.
   In incoherent gradient echo only the FID is sampled.
   In SSFP only the spin echo is sampled.
7. a

Chapter 6

1. When a nucleus only receives one pulse, i.e. either the 90° or the 180° pulse.
2. Because gradient rephasing is not slice selective so that all the spins that have been excited will be rephased and produce a signal.
3. Co-current.
4. b
5. Produce a signal void so that unwanted signal from flowing nuclei entering the FOV is nulled. Volumes should be placed inferiorally and on the right to null signal coming up the arm and from the chest.
6. To reduce flow artefact and to give flowing nuclei a bright signal.

Chapter 7

1. This is caused by under sampling of data in the phase direction. The system does not have sufficient data to encode low and high signal boundaries correctly. Increase phase encodings or NEX to remedy.
2. Magnetic susceptibility artefact. Always scan using spin echo pulse sequences.
3. Chemical shift occurs in frequency axis. Increased at high field strengths and when using reduced receive bandwidths. Chemical misregistration occurs along the phase axis and is increased when using gradient echo sequences and a TE that regenerates an echo when fat and water are out of phase.
4. When anatomy that is producing signal occurs outside the FOV in the phase direction.
5. (a) The incremental step between phase encodes is halved which doubles the FOV in the phase direction and doubles the number of phase encodes performed. Data is therefore over-sampled and only the middle portion of the FOV is displayed. The NEX is halved to maintain the scan time.
   (b) Each line of K space is filled randomly depending on chest motion. The central lines of K space are filled when the chest wall motion is at a minimum and the outer lines when the chest wall motion is at a maximum. In this way most of the signal and contrast is acquired when chest wall motion is minimised.
6. Cross talk occurs when energy is given up to nuclei in adjacent slices during relaxation. Cross excitation is caused by RF pulses exciting nuclei in adjacent slices. Only this can be compensated for by having a gap between slices, squaring the RF pulses off so that they fit the slices or by interleaving the slice acquisition.
7. Respiratory compensation, increasing NEX, gating, gradient moment rephasing, pre-saturation, breath-holding techniques, compression.

Chapter 8

1. False.
2. b
3. a
4. b
5. c
6. To give the system time to wait for the next R wave.
7. $800 - (80 + 4) = 716$ ms.
8. (a) Peripheral.
   (b) None.
   (c) Peripheral.
   (d) ECG.

Chapter 9

1. c	5. c
2. a	6. d
3. d	7. d
4. a	

Chapter 10

1. c	6. c
2. c	7. d
3. d	8. a
4. a	9. b
5. b	

Chapter 11

1. d	7. b
2. b	8. a
3. T1 and T2.	9. Pituitary adenoma.
4. Paramagnetic.	Post operative lumbar disc.
5. d	Liver lesions.
6. c	Breast imaging.

Chapter 12

1. d	5. d
2. a	6. a
3. d	7. b
4. b	8. c

Index

Note: MR images are indicated by italics.